Oxford American Handbook of
Reproductive Medicine

About the Oxford American Handbooks in Medicine

The Oxford American Handbooks are pocket clinical books, providing practical guidance in quick reference, note form. Titles cover major medical specialties or cross-specialty topics and are aimed at students, residents, internists, family physicians, and practicing physicians within specific disciplines.

Their reputation is built on including the best clinical information, complemented by hints, tips, and advice from the authors. Each one is carefully reviewed by senior subject experts, residents, and students to ensure that content reflects the reality of day-to-day medical practice.

Key series features

- Written in short chunks, each topic is covered in a two-page spread to enable readers to find information quickly. They are also perfect for test preparation and gaining a quick overview of a subject without scanning through unnecessary pages.
- Content is evidence based and complemented by the expertise and judgment of experienced authors.
- The Handbooks provide a humanistic approach to medicine—it's more than just treatment by numbers.
- A "friend in your pocket," the Handbooks offer honest, reliable guidance about the difficulties of practicing medicine and provide coverage of both the practice and art of medicine.
- For quick reference, useful "everyday" information is included on the inside covers.

Published and Forthcoming Oxford American Handbooks

Oxford American Handbook of Clinical Medicine
Oxford American Handbook of Anesthesiology
Oxford American Handbook of Cardiology
Oxford American Handbook of Clinical Dentistry
Oxford American Handbook of Clinical Diagnosis
Oxford American Handbook of Clinical Examination and Practical Skills
Oxford American Handbook of Clinical Pharmacy
Oxford American Handbook of Critical Care
Oxford American Handbook of Emergency Medicine
Oxford American Handbook of Endocrinology and Diabetes
Oxford American Handbook of Gastroenterology and Hepatology
Oxford American Handbook of Geriatric Medicine
Oxford American Handbook of Hospice and Palliative Medicine
Oxford American Handbook of Infectious Diseases
Oxford American Handbook of Nephrology and Hypertension
Oxford American Handbook of Neurology
Oxford American Handbook of Obstetrics and Gynecology
Oxford American Handbook of Oncology
Oxford American Handbook of Ophthalmology
Oxford American Handbook of Otolaryngology
Oxford American Handbook of Pediatrics
Oxford American Handbook of Physical Medicine and Rehabilitation
Oxford American Handbook of Psychiatry
Oxford American Handbook of Pulmonary Medicine
Oxford American Handbook of Reproductive Medicine
Oxford American Handbook of Rheumatology
Oxford American Handbook of Sports Medicine
Oxford American Handbook of Surgery
Oxford American Handbook of Urology

Oxford American Handbook of Reproductive Medicine

Hugh S. Taylor, MD
Professor and Director
Division of Reproductive
Endocrinology and Infertility
Yale University School of Medicine
New Haven, Connecticut

Tamir S. Aldad, MS-III
Predoctoral Research Fellow
Division of Reproductive
Endocrinology and Infertility
Yale University School of Medicine
New Haven, Connecticut

Enda McVeigh, FRCOG
Medical Director,
Oxford Fertility Unit, UK

Roy Homburg, FRCOG
Professor of Reproductive Medicine
Free University of Amsterdam,
Netherlands
and
Professor of Obstetrics &
Gynecology
Tel Aviv University, Israel

John Guillebaud, FRCSEd, FRCOG
Emeritus Professor of Family
Planning and
Reproductive Health
University College London, UK

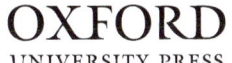

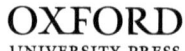
UNIVERSITY PRESS

Oxford University Press, Inc. publishes works that further
Oxford University's objective of excellence
in research, scholarship and education.

Oxford New York

Auckland Cape Town Dar es Salaam Hong Kong Karachi
Kuala Lumpur Madrid Melbourne Mexico City Nairobi
New Delhi Shanghai Taipei Toronto

With offices in

Argentina Austria Brazil Chile Czech Republic France Greece
Guatemala Hungary Italy Japan Poland Portugal
Singapore South Korea Switzerland Thailand Turkey Ukraine Vietnam

Copyright © 2012 by Oxford University Press, Inc.

Published by Oxford University Press Inc.
198 Madison Avenue, New York, New York 10016

www.oup.com

Oxford is a registered trademark of Oxford University Press

First published 2012

UK version published: 2008

All rights reserved. No part of this publication may be reproduced,
stored in a retrieval system, or transmitted, in any form or by any means,
electronic, mechanical, photocopying, recording, or otherwise,
without the prior permission of Oxford University Press.

Library of Congress Cataloging-in-Publication Data

Oxford American handbook of reproductive medicine / Hugh S. Taylor ... [et al.].
p. ; cm. — (Oxford American handbooks)
American handbook of reproductive medicine
Handbook of reproductive medicine
Includes index.
ISBN 978–0–19–973576–1
I. Taylor, Hugh S. II. Title: American handbook of reproductive medicine. III. Title:
Handbook of reproductive medicine. IV. Series: Oxford American handbooks.
[DNLM: 1. Reproductive Medicine—Handbooks. 2. Contraception—Handbooks. 3. Family
Planning Services—Handbooks. 4. Reproductive Techniques—Handbooks. WQ 39]

362.196'65—dc23
2011039715

This material is not intended to be, and should not be considered, a substitute for medical or other professional advice. Treatment for the conditions described in this material is highly dependent on the individual circumstances. And, while this material is designed to offer accurate information with respect to the subject matter covered and to be current as of the time it was written, research and knowledge about medical and health issues are constantly evolving and dose schedules for medications are being revised continually, with new side effects recognized and accounted for regularly. Readers must therefore always check the product information and clinical procedures with the most up-to-date published product information and data sheets provided by the manufacturers and the most recent codes of conduct and safety regulation. Oxford University Press and the authors make no representations or warranties to readers, express or implied, as to the accuracy or completeness of this material, including without limitation that they make no representation or warranties as to the accuracy or efficacy of the drug dosages mentioned in the material. The authors and the publishers do not accept, and expressly disclaim, any responsibility for any liability, loss, or risk that may be claimed or incurred as a consequence of the use and/or application of any of the contents of this material.

Preface

Welcome to the American edition of the *Oxford Handbook of Reproductive Medicine*. We have attempted to retain the fundamentals of the original handbook while adapting the text to an American audience and incorporating recent advances in obstetrics, gynecology, and reproductive medicine.

Reproductive medicine has seen major advancements in the last several years and continues to be at the forefront of medical research. In this Handbook, we provide a moderately comprehensive understanding of reproductive medicine by discussing male and female reproductive physiology, presenting common diseases, and providing different management options. Many factors can affect reproduction; thus we have included clear and concise algorithms focusing on puberty, the menstrual cycle, and infertility that can quickly and easily be reviewed prior to diagnosing and managing a patient. We have emphasized particularly the most commonly seen pathologies and their standard of care, as we hope that this book will be used as a day-to-day reference. The second portion of the handbook discusses contraception and the options currently available in the United States. We have included the advantages and disadvantages of each, to provide a conveniently organized reference when one is answering questions commonly asked by patients.

This Handbook is a valuable resource for trainees, students, and clinicians. We hope that the *Oxford American Handbook of Reproductive Medicine* will be an essential addition to your personal library and provide you with concise, easily interpreted information that you can effortlessly incorporate into your studies and professional practice.

Hugh S. Taylor
Tamir S. Aldad

Acknowledgments

The editors of the *Oxford American Handbook of Reproductive Medicine* would like to thank the authors of the original UK version of the Oxford Handbook as well as the editorial staff at Oxford University Press in New York for their commitment, hard work, and unconditional effort throughout the editorial process. We would also like to thank our families, friends, and fellow colleagues for their support and encouragement.

Contents

Detailed contents *xiii*
Symbols and abbreviations *xxi*

Part 1: Reproductive Medicine

1	Sexual differentiation	3
2	Steroid hormones	15
3	Menarche and adolescent gynecology	23
4	Ovaries and the menstrual cycle	31
5	Polycystic ovary syndrome	41
6	Hirsutism and virilization	51
7	Amenorrhea and oligomenorrhea	61
8	Menopause and hormone replacement therapy	73
9	Initial advice regarding delays in conception	83
10	Defining infertility	87
11	Investigation of fertility problems	91
12	Management strategies for fertility problems	103
13	Male infertility	111
14	Ovulation induction	121
15	Tubal and uterine disorders	135
16	Medical and surgical management of endometriosis	141
17	Intrauterine insemination	151
18	In vitro fertilization (IVF) and associated assisted conception techniques	155

Part 2: Contraception and Family Planning

19	Fertility and fertility awareness	169
20	Male contraception	181

21	Vaginal methods	**187**
22	The combined oral contraceptive (COC)	**193**
23	The progestogen-only pill (POP)	**223**
24	Injectables	**231**
25	Contraceptive implants	**239**
26	Intrauterine contraception	**247**
27	Postcoital contraception	**261**
28	Sterilization	**269**
29	Special considerations	**275**
	Appendix	**281**

Index *283*

Detailed contents

Symbols and abbreviations *xxi*

1 Sexual differentiation — 3

Key stages of fetal sex differentiation *4*
The SRY gene *5*
Other genes involved in sex determination *6*
Abnormal embryological development—intersex conditions *7*
Hermaphroditism *9*
Müllerian anomalies *10*
Hand–foot–genital syndrome *12*
Incomplete regression of the Wolffian system *13*

2 Steroid hormones — 15

Introduction *16*
Steroid hormone biosynthesis reactions *18*
Gonadal steroid hormones *21*
Steroid-binding proteins *22*
Further reading *22*

3 Menarche and adolescent gynecology — 23

Introduction *24*
Hypothalamic–pituitary–gonadal axis *25*
Stages of puberty *27*
Precocious puberty *28*
Delayed puberty *29*
Further reading *30*

4 Ovaries and the menstrual cycle — 31

Introduction *32*
Hormones *34*
The ovary *36*
Follicular development *37*
Causes of anovulation and oligo-ovulation *38*

5 Polycystic ovary syndrome — 41

Introduction 42
Definition 43
Prevalence 44
Etiology 44
Pathophysiology 45
Management 47
Long-term health implications of PCOS 50
Further reading 50

6 Hirsutism and virilization — 51

Introduction 52
Pathophysiology 53
History and examination 54
Etiology 55
Differential diagnosis 56
Treatment 58

7 Amenorrhea and oligomenorrhea — 61

Introduction 62
Etiology 63
Investigations 67
Management 70

8 Menopause and hormone replacement therapy — 73

Introduction 74
Pathophysiology 74
Other hormonal changes 75
Symptoms 75
Women's Health Initiative (WHI) trial 79
Risks and benefits of HRT 80
HRT preparations 81
Alternative treatment 82

9 Initial regarding delays in conception — 83

Prevalence of fertility problems 84
Timing of the initial investigation 84

Female partner's age 85
Frequency and timing of intercourse 85
Environmental and dietary influences 86

10 Defining infertility   87

Introduction 88
General points before starting investigation 89

11 Investigation of fertility problems   91

Introduction 92
Investigation of the male partner 95
Investigation of the female partner 98
Investigation of a possible mechanical factor 100
Further reading 102

12 Management strategies for fertility problems   103

Principles 104
Management of investigations 105
Management strategies 106

13 Male infertility   111

Introduction 112
Etiology 113
Investigation of the male 116
Further reading and information 120

14 Ovulation induction   121

Introduction 122
Clomifene citrate 123
Aromatase inhibitors 125
Metformin 126
Pulsatile gonadotropin-releasing hormone (gonadorelin) 127
Gonadotropins 128
Laparoscopic ovarian drilling (LOD) 133
Further reading 133

15 Tubal and uterine disorders — 135

Introduction *136*
Tubal disorders *137*
Surgery to the fallopian tube *139*
Uterine disorders *140*

16 Medical and surgical management of endometriosis — 141

Introduction *142*
Examination and investigations *143*
Endometriosis-associated infertility *144*
Surgical treatment of endometriosis *145*
Principles of surgery for infertility patients with endometriosis *147*
Medical treatment *148*
Further reading and information *150*

17 Intrauterine insemination — 151

Introduction *152*
Methods *152*
Principle *152*
Indications *153*
IUI for mild male-factor infertility *153*
IUI for unexplained infertility *153*
Cost-effectiveness *154*
Conclusions *154*
Further reading *154*

18 In vitro fertilization and associated assisted conception techniques — 155

Introduction *156*
Factors affecting the outcome of IVF *157*
Number of embryos transferred *158*
Procedures used during IVF *159*
Intracytoplasmic sperm injection *163*
Oocyte donation *163*
Complications of IVF *164*
Preimplantation genetic diagnosis (PGD)/preimplantation genetic screening (PGS) *165*

Follow-up of children born as a result of assisted reproduction *166*
Further reading and information *166*

19 Fertility and fertility awareness 169

Introduction *170*
Sex and relationships education (SRE) *170*
Sexually transmitted infections *171*
Features of the ideal contraceptive *172*
Relative effectiveness of the available methods *173*
Eligibility criteria for contraceptives *175*
Fertility awareness and methods for the natural regulation of fertility *176*

20 Male contraception 181

Coitus interruptus *182*
Male condoms *183*
The male pill *184*
Vasectomy *185*

21 Vaginal methods 187

Female condoms *188*
Caps and diaphragms *189*
Spermicide (nonoxinol) *190*

22 The combined oral contraceptive (COC) 193

Mechanism of action *194*
Benefits versus risks *195*
Tumor risk and COCs *196*
Cardiovascular disease *199*
Eligibility criteria for COCs *205*
The pill-free interval (PFI) *000*
Drug interactions *212*
Other relevant drugs *213*
Counseling and ongoing supervision *216*
Stopping COCs *220*
Other combined methods *221*
Pill follow-up *221*
Congenital abnormalities and fertility issues *222*

23 The progestogen-only pill (POP) — 223

Mechanism of action and maintenance of effectiveness 224
Risks and disadvantages 225
Advantages and indications 226
Problems and contraindications 227
Counseling and ongoing supervision 228

24 Injectables — 231

Introduction 232
Mechanism of action and effectiveness 233
Indications 234
Advantages 234
Problems and disadvantages 235
Contraindications 237
Counseling and ongoing supervision 238

25 Contraceptive implants — 239

Introduction 240
Mechanism of action, administration, and effectiveness 241
Enzyme inducer drug (EID) treatment 242
Reversibility and removal problems 242
Indications 243
Advantages 243
Disadvantages and contraindications 244
Counseling and ongoing supervision 245

26 Intrauterine contraception — 247

Introduction 248
Copper-bearing devices 249
The levonorgestrel-releasing intrauterine system (LNG-IUS) 255

27 Postcoital contraception — 261

Introduction 262
Levonorgestrel emergency contraception (LNG-EC) 263
Copper intrauterine devices (IUDs) 264
Counseling and management 265
Special indications for EC 267

28 Sterilization — 269

Introduction 270
Efficacy considerations 271
Potential reversibility 272
Possible long-term side effects of female sterilization 273
Comparison of methods 274

29 Special considerations — 275

How can a provider be reasonably sure of a woman not being pregnant? 276
Contraception at the climacteric 278

Appendix — 281

Essential Web sites in reproductive health 282
Further reading and references 282

Index 283

Symbols and abbreviations

♣	controversial topic
📖	page number in this volume
ABP	androgen-binding protein
ACTH	adrenocorticotropic hormone
ACOG	American College of Obstetrics and Gynecology
AFS	American Fertility Society
ALO	*Actinomyces*-like organisms
AMH	anti-Müllerian hormone
AMI	acute myocardial infarction
AP	anterposterior
ART	assisted reproductive technologies
ASRM	American Society for Reproductive Medicine
BBD	benign breast disease
BBT	basal body temperature
bid	twice a day
BMI	body mass index
BP	blood pressure
BTB	breakthrough bleeding
CAH	congenital adrenal hyperplasia
CAIS	complete androgen insensitivity syndrome
CBG	corticosteroid-binding globulin
CC	clomifene citrate
CHD	coronary heart disease
CIN	cervical intraepithelial neoplasia
CNS	central nervous system
COC	combined oral contraception or contraceptive
COEC	combined oral emergency contraceptive
CPA	cyproterone acetate
CRH	corticotropin-releasing hormone
CT	computed tomography
CVS	cardiovascular system
DES	diethylstilboestrol
DHEAS	dehydroepiandosterone sulfate
DHT	dihydrotestosterone
DM	diabetes mellitus
DMPA	depot medroxyprogesterone acetate
DSG	desogestrel
DSP	drospirenone

DVT	deep venous thrombosis
EC	emergency contraception
EE	ethinylestradiol
EGF	epidermal growth factor
EID	enzyme inducer drug
ERT	estrogen replacement therapy
ESHRE	European Society for Human Reproduction
ET	embryo transfer
EVA	ethylene vinyl acetate
FAQ	frequently asked question
FDA	Food and Drug Administration
FERC	frozen embryo replacement cycle
FSH	follicle-stimulating hormone
GBG	gonadal steroid-binding globulin
GIFT	gamete intrafallopian tube transfer
GnRH	gonadotropin-releasing hormone
GSD	gestodene
GUM	genitourinary medicine
hCG	human chorionic gonadotropin
HDL	high-density lipoprotein
HFG	hand–foot–genital (syndrome)
HIV	human immunodeficiency virus
hMG	human menopausal gonadotropin
HMG	high-mobility group
HPV	human papillomavirus
HRT	hormone replacement therapy
HS	hemorrhagic stroke
HSG	hysterosalpingography
5-HT	5-hydroxytryptamine
HUS	hemolytic uremic syndrome
ICSI	intracytoplasmic sperm injection
IM	intramuscular
INR	international normalized ratio
IS	ischemic stroke
IUD	intrauterine device
IUI	intrauterine insemination
IUS	intrauterine system
IV	intravenous
IVF	in vitro fertilization
LAM	lactational amenorrhea method
LARC	long-acting reversible contraceptive

LCR	ligase chain reaction—ultrasensitive and specific test (e.g., for chlamydia)
LDL	low-density lipoprotein
LH	luteinizing hormone
LNG	levonorgestrel
LOCAH	late-onset congenital adrenal hyperplasia
LOD	laparoscopic ovarian drilling
MAO	monamine oxidase
MAR	mixed antibody reaction
MESA	microsurgical epididymal sperm aspiration
MIS	Müllerian-inhibiting substance
MPA	medroxyprogesterone acetate
MRI	magnetic resonance imaging
MRKH	Mayer–Rokitansky–Kuster–Hauser
NET	norethindrone
NETA	norethisterone acetate
NGM	norgestimate
NICHD	National Institute of Child Health & Human Development
NIH	National Institutes of Health
OC	oral contraceptive
OHSS	ovarian hyperstimulation syndrome
OR	odds ratio
PCOS	polycystic ovarian syndrome
PCR	polymerase chain reaction
PCT	postcoital test
PE	pulmonary embolism
PESA	percutaneous epididymal sperm aspiration
PFI	pill-free interval
PID	pelvic inflammatory disease
PKC	protein kinase C
PMS	premenstrual syndrome
POEC	progestogen-only emergency contraceptive
POP	progestogen-only pill
RCT	randomized controlled trial
SART	Society for Assisted Reproductive Medicine
SC	subcutaneous
SD	standard deviation
SHGB	sex hormone–binding globulin
SLE	systemic lupus erythematosus
SPC	summary of product characteristics
SRE	sex and relationships education

S/S	saline-infused sonohistogram
STD	sexually transmitted disease
TESE	testicular sperm extraction
TGF	transforming growth factor
TIA	transient ischemic attack
TSH	thyroid-stimulating hormone
TTP	thrombotic thrombocytopenic purpura
TVS	transvaginal scanning
UPSI	unprotected sexual intercourse
VTE	venous thromboembolism
VV	varicose veins
WHI	Women's Health Initiative
WHO	World Health Organization
WHOMEC	WHO Medical Eligibility Criteria (for contraceptive use)
WHOSPR	WHO Selected Practice Recommendations (for contraceptive use)

Part 1

Reproductive Medicine

1 Sexual differentiation	**3**
2 Steroid hormones	**15**
3 Menarche and adolescent gynecology	**23**
4 Ovaries and the menstrual cycle	**31**
5 Polycystic ovary syndrome	**41**
6 Hirsutism and virilization	**51**
7 Amenorrhea and oligomenorrhea	**61**
8 Menopause and hormone replacement therapy	**73**
9 Initial advice regarding delays in conception	**83**
10 Defining infertility	**87**
11 Investigation of fertility problems	**91**
12 Management strategies for fertility problems	**103**
13 Male infertility	**111**
14 Ovulation induction	**121**
15 Tubal and uterine disorders	**135**
16 Medical and surgical management of endometriosis	**141**
17 Intrauterine insemination	**151**
18 In vitro fertilization (IVF) and associated assisted conception techniques	**155**

Chapter 1

Sexual differentiation

Key stages of fetal sex differentiation *4*
The SRY gene *5*
Other genes involved in sex determination *6*
Abnormal embryological development—intersex conditions *7*
Hermaphroditism *9*
Müllerian anomalies *10*
Hand–foot–genital syndrome *12*
Incomplete regression of the Wolffian system *13*

Key stages of fetal sex differentiation

Genetic sex is determined at the moment of conception by the presence or absence of the Y chromosome. After week 6 of fetal life, it will guide the subsequent development of the fetus down one of two standard pathways—male or female (see Fig. 1.1).

- Week 3: Primordial germ cells present in the endoderm of the yolk sac.
- Week 5–6: Germs cells migrate to the genital ridge (future gonad).
- Week 6: Primitive sex cords form around the germ cells—two Müllerian (or paramesonephric) ducts lateral to the Wolffian (or mesonephric) ducts.
- Week 6: The cloacal membrane at the caudal end of the fetus separates into the anterior urogenital and posterior anal parts.
- Week 7: The urogenital section of the cloacal membrane, the genital tubercle, urogenital folds, and lateral and labioscrotal swelling will differentiate into the future external genitalia.

After gonadal differentiation has occurred, the presence or absence of gonadal hormone production and other fetal factors then guides development of the Müllerian ducts, Wolffian ducts, and external genitalia.

The testes secrete androgens, leading to male external genital development and differentiation of the bilateral Wolffian ducts into the vas deferens, seminal vesicle, and epididymis. The testes also secrete anti-Müllerian hormone (AMH—also know as Müllerian-inhibiting substance, MIS), leading to the regression of the Müllerian ducts.

The fetal ovaries do not secrete androgens or AMH and therefore the female external genital development, growth of the Müllerian ducts and spontaneous regression of the Wolffian ducts occur.

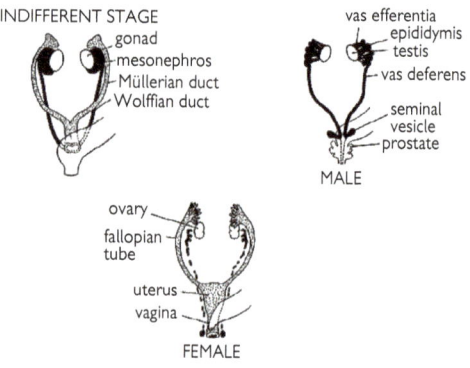

Figure 1.1 Key stages of fetal sex differentiation.

Box 1.1 Development of the female reproductive system
- Gonads are undifferentiated until 7–8 weeks of gestation.
- Differentiation is associated with a dual ductal system.
- Mesonephric ducts form first.
- At 6 weeks, paramesonephric ducts form lateral to the mesonephric ducts.
- Mesonephric ducts degenerate.
- Müllerian ducts form.
  - Cranial ends become fallopian tubes.
  - Caudal ends fuse to form the uterus, cervix, and upper vagina.
- By ~9 weeks, a uterine cervix is visible.
- By 17 weeks, myometrium is formed.

The *SRY* gene

The presence or absence of the *SRY* gene (sex-determining region of the Y chromosome) at the end of week 6 of fetal development will guide the undifferentiated gonad to commence development into an ovary or testis.

Key facts about the *SRY* gene include the following:
- High-mobility group (HMG) box family of DNA-binding proteins
- Master control gene for testis determination
- DNA/RNA-binding protein
- Molecular targets unknown
- Precipitates cascade of gene expression required for testis formation
- Expression is transiently activated in a center-to-pole wave along the anteroposterior (AP) axis of developing XY gonads.
- Shortly after the onset of *Sry* activation, *Sox9* (*Sry*-related HMG box-9) is also activated in a center-to-pole pattern similar to the initial *Sry* expression profile.

Other genes involved in sex determination

There are two other genes, *DMRT1* and *DAX1*, that are involved in sex determination in the developing fetus.

DMRT1
- Chromosome 9 transcription factor
- Critical in human sex determination—expressed in genital ridges and in Sertoli cells. It increases during testis development and decreases in the ovary.
- Mutations in this region are associated with male-to-female sex reversal.
- *DMT1*-related sequences have also been found in the chick, alligator, and mouse.
- *DMRT* genes are expressed only in the genital ridges of male embryos.

DAX1
- Chromosome X p21.3–p21.2 nuclear receptor family
- Expressed in both gonadal ridges, then persists in the ovary and decreases in the testis according to switch on of *Sry*
- Anti-testis gene by acting antagonistically to *Sry*?
- Responsible for DSS syndrome (dosage-sensitive sex reversal). Dosage-sensitive sex reversal is due to duplication of the gene in humans.

Abnormal embryological development—intersex conditions

Intersex is defined as a mix or blend of the physically defining features associated with the male or females, i.e., karyotype, gonadal structure, internal genitalia, and external genitalia.

Most intersex conditions occur from a genetic or environmental disruption to the pathway of fetal sexual development. This disruption can be to gonadal differentiation or development, sex steroid production, sex steroid conversion, or tissue utilization of sex steroid.

Incidence

The estimated incidence in the United States is 1 in 2000. Conditions with autosomal recessive inheritance are more common in populations in which intermarriage is common.

Presentation and investigation

Each intersex condition has a spectrum of severity and therefore may present in a variety of ways:

- Ambiguous genitalia
- Salt-losing crisis in neonatal life (congenital adrenal hyperplasia)
- Pelvic mass with gonadal tumor
- Inguinal hernia with unexpected gonad
- Ambiguity of the genitalia developing in childhood or puberty
- Sibling history of intersex
- Primary amenorrhea or puberty delay
- Infertility
- Sexual dysfunction

Initial investigation will depend on the presentation but should include those listed in Table 1.1.

Table 1.1 Investigations for intersex conditions.

Initial investigation	Further investigations
Karyotype	Androstendione
Testosterone and estradiol	Dihydrotestosterone (DHT)
Luteinizing hormone (LH) and follicle-stimulating hormone (FSH)	24-hour urine for steroid metabolites
17-Hydroxyprogesterone	Synacthen test
Pelvic imaging—ultrasound or MRI	Renal ultrasound

Management of intersex conditions

The management of these conditions will depend on acquiring an accurate diagnosis and then referral to an appropriate pediatric or adult multidisciplinary team (endocrinology, gynecology, surgery, and psychology). Areas that the team will have to consider include the following:
- Need for hormone replacement
- Screening for associated medical conditions
- Psychological treatment
- Genetic counseling for other family members
- Sex assignment for children
- Gonadal malignancy risk
- Fertility options
- Genital surgery options for ambiguous genitalia
- Vaginal enlargement options
- Access to peer support

The disorders can be categorized into three main areas: gonadal dysgenesis (complete and partial), hermaphroditism (true/primary and pseudo/secondary), and dysgenesis of the uterus, vagina, and external genitalia.

Complete (pure) gonadal dysgenesis
This is due to a primary defect in gonadal formation. The karyotype may be a normal 46, XX or 46, XY.

Little is known about the 46, XX condition apart from the fact that some individuals have homozygous FSH receptor mutations, also seen in males when they have impaired spermatogenesis.

In the 46, XY condition, 20% have lesions in the *SRY* gene, while the remainder have the abnormalities in the X chromosome or autosomes. In these cases, gonadal development is arrested before MIS (AMH) and androgens are produced. This results in formation of bilateral streak gonads associated with an immature female phenotype. There are no other associated somatic defects.

The result clinically is a delayed puberty and amenorrhea, which is estrogen responsive.

Complete gonadal dysgenesis
This condition is also the result of a primary defect in gonadal formation, but in these cases there are bilateral streak gonads. Typically, the karotype is 45, XO Turner's syndrome, and all patients have partial or complete loss of material from an X chromosome.

It occurs in 1 in 2500 live births. Somatic defects are present in these cases and include facial dystrophy, short stature, and renal anomalies.

There is a delay in puberty which is estrogen responsive. Fertility is rare but is reported more in cases of mosaicism.

Mixed gonadal dysgenesis
This occurs in mosaics: 46, XY or 45 XO; 46, XY. It results in unilateral testis and contralateral streak gonad. There is persistence of the Müllerian duct structures, the vagina, and uterus, and most individuals have a fallopian tube on the side of the streak. The external genitalia are ambiguous. In the case of XY, they are undervirilized.

Hermaphroditism

Hermaphroditism is defined as "true" in cases where there is both an ovary and testis or an ovotestis, or as pseudohermaphrodite (male) where there are two testes and pseudohermaphrodite (female) where there are two ovaries.

The most common karyotype in true hermaphroditism is 46, XX. Ovarian and testicular tissues can be present separately or as an ovotestis. The external genitalia tend to be masculinized.

Secondary or pseudohermaphrodites

(XY) Testicular feminization or androgen insensitivity syndrome occurs. Complete = testis + female soma, with a population incidence of 0.005%; partial = poorly developed male soma, with population incidence of 0.01%. There is a defect in the androgen receptor or in androgen synthesis.

Affected individuals have MIS; thus no Müllerian ducts or associated structures develop. In complete androgen insensitivity syndrome (CAIS), there can be completely normal external genitalia.

Absent or rudimentary Wolffian duct derivatives occur, with an absence or presence of epididymides and/or vas deferens. Inguinal or labial testes are present and a short, blind-ending vagina.

(XX) Congenital adrenohyperplasia or adrenogenital syndrome comprises presence of an ovary + variable somatic maleness; the partial form has a population incidence of 1%, the complete form, 0.01%.

21-Hydroxylase deficiency is the most common autosomal recessive genetic disorder. It is the most common cause of genital ambiguity of the newborn in the United States.

The genitalia can range from clitoral enlargement to complete labioscrotal fusion and a penile urethra. The size and entry level of vagina into the urogenital sinus are abnormal. There are normal internal Müllerian duct derivatives. An increase in androgens can be seen as early as 7–8 weeks of fetal life, but there is no MIS.

(XY) 5-alpha-reductase deficiency involves 46, XY individuals with normal testes but lacking the enzyme in external genitalia and urogenital sinus and unable to make DHT. They are minimally virilized at birth then experience extreme virilization at puberty.

Müllerian anomalies

Abnormal development of the Müllerian ducts can lead to a wide range of conditions. Many are subtle variations of normal Müllerian anatomy and often remain asymptomatic or require no treatment. Others are transverse or longitudinal structures and may present in a variety of ways.

An understanding of the timing and sequence of embryological development of the entire urogenital system helps toward understanding the conditions (see Fig. 1.2).

- Vaginal development begins at 9 weeks.
- Uterovaginal plate forms between the caudal buds of the Müllerian ducts and dorsal wall of the urogenital sinus.
- Approximately 1/3 of vagina develops from paramesonephric ducts.
- Remainder from urogenital sinus.

Müllerian anomalies—The American Society for Reproductive Medicine (ASRM) classification

The classification most used to list Müllerian anomalies is that of the American Society for Reproductive Medicine. Congenital Müllerian

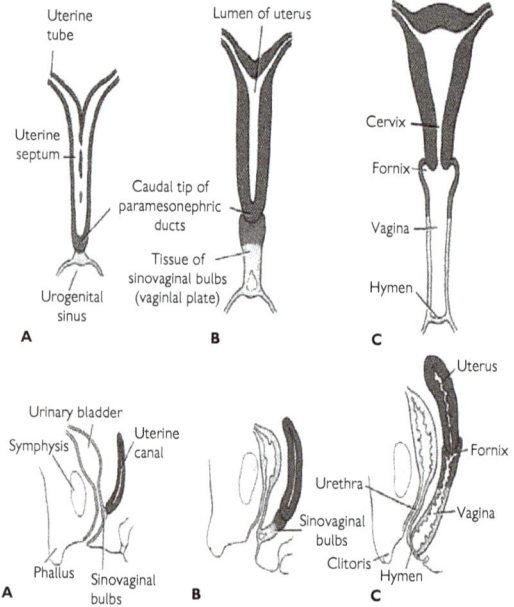

Figure 1.2 Normal Müllerian development.

abnormalities generally fall into one of three groups: a normally fused single Müllerian system with agenesis of one or more parts; a unicornuate system (unilateral hypoplasia or agenesis of one Müllerian dust); or lateral fusion failures (including didelphic and bicornuate anomalies) (Fig. 1.3).

Complete agenesis is separated in Rokitansky syndrome (also called Mayer–Rokitansky–Kuster–Hauser [MRKH] syndrome).

- Class I (hypoplasia/agenesis): uterine or cervical agenesis or hypoplasia. MRKH syndrome involves combined agenesis of the uterus, cervix, and upper portion of the vagina.
- Class II (unicornuate uterus): a unicornuate uterus is the result of complete, or almost complete, arrest of development of one Müllerian duct. It is incomplete in 90% of patients.

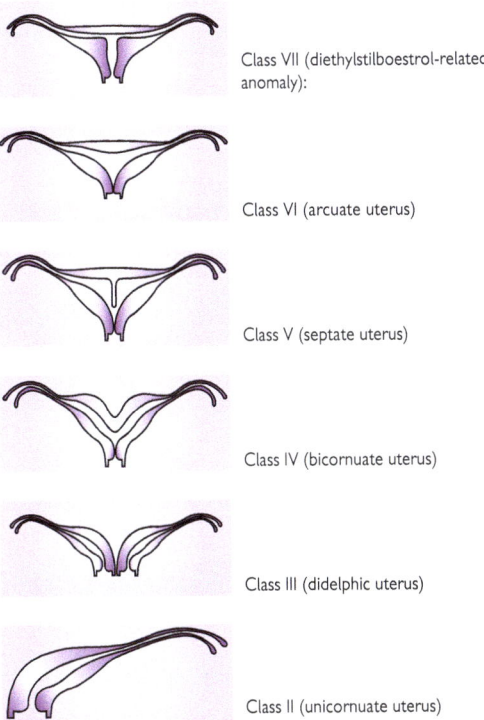

Class VII (diethylstilboestrol-related anomaly):

Class VI (arcuate uterus)

Class V (septate uterus)

Class IV (bicornuate uterus)

Class III (didelphic uterus)

Class II (unicornuate uterus)

Figure 1.3 The American Society for Reproductive Medicine (ASRM) classification of Müllerian anomalies.

- Class III (didelphic uterus): complete non-fusion of both Müllerian ducts. The individual horns are fully developed and almost normal in size. There are two cervices.
- Class IV (bicornuate uterus): partial non-fusion of the Müllerian ducts
- Class V (septate uterus): a septate uterus results from failure of resorption of the septum between the two uterine horns. The septum can be partial or complete.
- Class VI (arcuate uterus): an arcuate uterus has a single uterine cavity with a convex or flat uterine fundus.
- Class VII (diethylstilboestrol [DES]-related anomaly):
  - Seen in the female offspring of as many as 15% of women exposed to DES during pregnancy
  - Uterine hypoplasia
  - T-shaped uterine cavity
  - Abnormal transverse ridges
  - Stenoses of the cervix
  - Vaginal adenosis
  - Increased risk of vaginal clear cell carcinoma
  - Adverse pregnancy outcome

The American Society for Reproductive Medicine (ASRM) classification of Müllerian anomalies

Hand–foot–genital syndrome

The *HOX* gene directs the differential identity of segments of the Müllerian ducts into the fallopian tubes, uterus, cervix, and upper vagina.

Hand–foot–genital (HFG) syndrome is a very rare autosomal dominant condition that is a result of 7 p15–p14.2 mutations in the Hox13A gene. It leads to skeletal anomalies in distal limbs and urogenital abnormalities:
- Short, proximally placed thumbs with hypoplastic thenar eminences
- Ulnar deviation of the second finger
- Clinodactyly of the fifth finger
- Short, medially deviated hallucies
- Brachydactyly of the second to fifth toes
- Shortening of the carpals and tarsals
- Bicornuate uterus
- Vaginal septum
- Ectopic localization of ureteric and urethral orifices
- Vesicoureteric reflux and ureteropelvic obstruction have been observed in females as well as in males. Hypospadias occurs in some affected males.

Incomplete regression of the Wolffian system

Parts of the Wolffian ducts may fail to regress completely in females and present as cysts lateral to the Müllerian ducts. Usually they are incidental findings and most are asymptomatic.

The epoophoron and the paraoophoron can be found beside the ovary and the mesosalpinx. Cysts of Gartner's ducts (the lower part of the Wolffian ducts) can occur anywhere from the broad ligament down to the vagina and may present as vulval or vaginal masses.

Imaging of the renal tract should be performed whenever abnormalities of the Müllerian system are found.

Chapter 2

Steroid hormones

Introduction *16*
Steroid hormone biosynthesis reactions *18*
Gonadal steroid hormones *21*
Steroid-binding proteins *22*
Further reading *22*

CHAPTER 2 Steroid hormones

Introduction

Steroid hormones are synthesized mainly in the gonads (testis and ovary) and the adrenals and (during gestation) by the fetoplacental unit. They act on peripheral target tissues and the central nervous system (CNS).

Gonadal steroids influence the sexual differentiation of the genitalia and of the brain, determine secondary sexual characteristics during development and sexual maturation, contribute to the maintenance of their functional state in adulthood, and control or modulate sexual behavior.

There are five major classes of steroid hormones: the progestagens (progestational hormones), glucocorticoids (anti-stressing hormones), mineralocorticoids (Na+ uptake regulators), androgens (male sex hormones), and estrogens (female sex hormones).

Steroids are lipophilic, low-molecular-weight compounds derived from cholesterol, which contains a ring system (cyclopentanophenanthrene ring) that is not broken down in mammalian cells. Cholesterol (Fig. 2.1a) contains 27 carbons, all of which are derived from acetate.

Cholesterol, and each of the steroid hormones, has four rings designated A, B, C, and D. In steroid hormones, these rings are fused in a *trans*

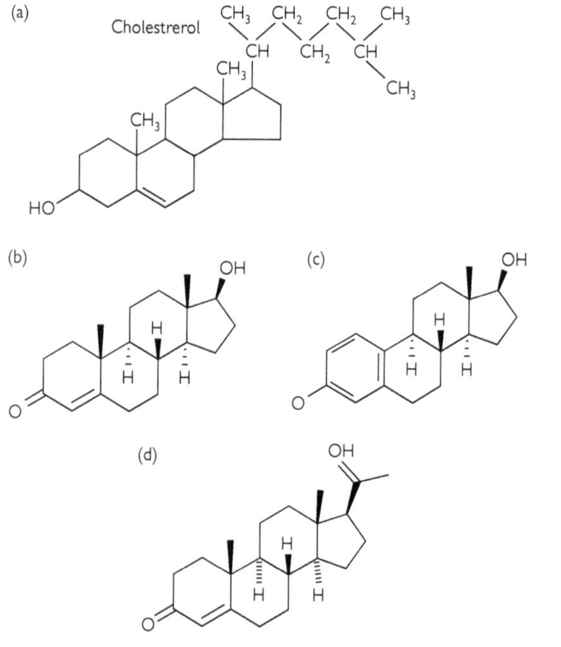

Figure 2.1 (a) Cholesterol, (b) Testosterone, (c) Estradiol, (d) Progesterone.

orientation to form an overall planar structure (unlike in bile acids, where they are in a *cis* formation leading to a curved structure).

The conversion of C27 cholesterol to the 18-, 19- and 21-carbon steroid hormones involves the rate-limiting, irreversible cleavage of a 6-carbon residue from cholesterol, producing pregnenolone (C21) plus isocaproaldehyde.

Steroids are extensively metabolized peripherally, notably in the liver, and in their target tissues, where conversion to an active form is sometimes required before they can elicit their biological responses. Steroid metabolism is therefore important not only for the production of these hormones but also for the regulation of their cellular and physiological actions.

Steroid hormone biosynthesis reactions

The particular steroid hormone class synthesized by a given cell type depends on its complement of peptide hormone receptors, its response to peptide hormone stimulation, and its genetically expressed complement of enzymes. Table 2.1 indicates the peptide hormone that is responsible for stimulating the synthesis of each steroid hormone.

The first reaction in converting cholesterol to C18, C19, and C21 steroids involves the cleavage of a 6-carbon group from cholesterol and is the principal committing, regulated, and rate-limiting step in steroid biosynthesis. The enzyme system that catalyses the cleavage reaction is known as P450-linked side chain-cleaving enzyme (P450ssc), or desmolase, and is found in the mitochondria of steroid-producing cells, but not in significant quantities in other cells.

Steroids of the adrenal cortex

The adrenal cortex is responsible for production of three major classes of steroid hormones: glucocorticoids, which regulate carbohydrate metabolism; mineralocorticoids, which regulate the body levels of sodium and potassium; and androgens, whose actions are similar to those of steroids produced by the male gonads (see Fig. 2.2).

Adrenal insufficiency is known as Addison disease, and in the absence of steroid hormone replacement therapy can rapidly cause death (in 1–2 weeks).

The adrenal cortex is composed of three main tissue regions: zona glomerulosa, zona fasciculata, and zona reticularis. Although the pathway to pregnenolone synthesis is the same in all zones of the cortex, the zones are histologically and enzymatically distinct, with the exact steroid hormone product dependent on the enzymes present in the cells of each zone.

Regulation of adrenal steroid synthesis

Adrenocorticotropic hormone (ACTH) of the hypothalamus regulates the hormone production of the zona fasciculata and zona reticularis. ACTH receptors in the plasma membrane activate adenylate cyclase with production of the second messenger, cAMP. The effect of ACTH on the production of cortisol is particularly important, with the result that a classic

Table 2.1 Peptide hormones and associated steroid hormones

Peptide hormone	Steroid hormone
Luteinizing hormone (LH)	Progesterone and testosterone
Adrenocorticotropic hormone (ACTH)	Cortisol
Follicle-stimulating hormone (FSH)	Estradiol
Angiotensin II/III	Aldosterone

STEROID HORMONE BIOSYNTHESIS REACTIONS

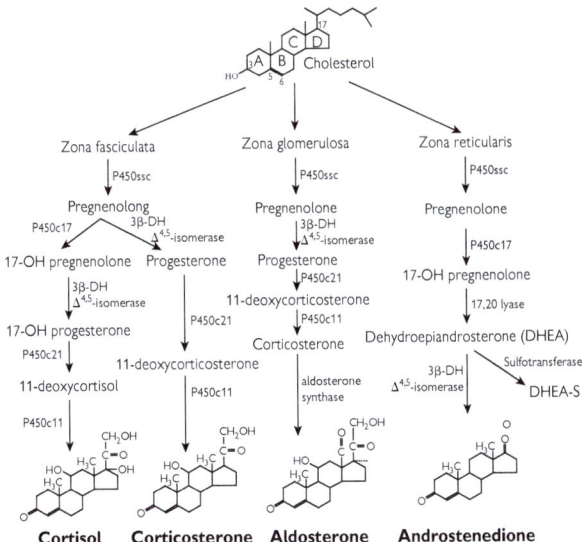

Figure 2.2 Synthesis of the various adrenal steroid hormones from cholesterol.

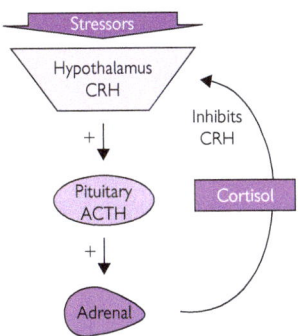

Figure 2.3 Feedback loop for the control of cortisol production.

feedback loop is prominent in regulating the circulating levels of corticotropin-releasing hormone (CRH), ACTH, and cortisol (Fig. 2.3).

Mineralocorticoid secretion from the zona glomerulosa is stimulated by an entirely different mechanism. Angiotensins II and III, derived from the action of the kidney protease renin on liver-derived angiotensinogen, stimulate zona glomerulosa cells by binding a plasma membrane receptor coupled to phospholipase C. Thus, angiotensin II and III binding to their receptor leads to the activation of protein kinase C (PKC) and elevated intracellular Ca^{2+} levels. These events lead to increased P450ssc activity and increased production of aldosterone.

In the kidney, aldosterone regulates sodium retention by stimulating gene expression of mRNA for the Na^+/K^+-ATPase responsible for the reaccumulation of sodium from the urine. The interplay between renin from the kidney and plasma angiotensinogen is important in regulating plasma aldosterone levels, sodium and potassium levels, and, ultimately, blood pressure.

Disorders resulting from defects in steroid biosynthesis

A number of endocrine disorders can be attributed to specific enzyme defects. Thus, inability to secrete normal levels of adrenal steroids may result in congenital adrenal hyperplasia (CAH) following hyperstimulation by ACTH (the negative steroid feedback controlling adrenal activity is lost).

In most cases, this syndrome is due to 21-hydroxylase deficiency and is associated with increased adrenal androgen secretion and partial virilization in girls.

Less common adrenal enzyme deficiencies involving either 17-hydroxylase (with a possible increase in mineralocorticoid levels) or 18-hydroxylase (aldosterone may be deficient with normal levels of cortisol) may occur.

Gonadal steroid hormones

The two most important steroids produced by the gonads are testosterone and estradiol (see Fig. 2.1b and 2.1c; 2.4). These compounds are under tight biosynthetic control, with short and long negative feedback loops that regulate the secretion of FSH and LH by the pituitary, and gonadotropin-releasing hormone (GnRH) by the hypothalamus.

The biosynthetic pathway to sex hormones in male and female gonadal tissue includes the production of the androgens—androstenedione and dehydroepiandrosterone. Testes and ovaries contain an additional enzyme, a 17-hydroxysteroid dehydrogenase, that enables androgens to be converted to testosterone.

In males, LH binds to Leydig cells, stimulating production of the principal Leydig cell hormone, testosterone. Testosterone is secreted to the plasma and also carried to Sertoli cells by androgen-binding protein (ABP). In Sertoli cells, the Δ-4 double bond of testosterone is reduced, producing dihydrotestosterone (DHT).

Testosterone and DHT are carried in the plasma and delivered to target tissue by a specific gonadal steroid-binding globulin (GBG). In a number of target tissues, testosterone can be converted to DHT.

DHT is the most potent of the male steroid hormones, with an activity that is 10 times that of testosterone. Because of its relatively lower potency, testosterone is sometimes considered to be a prohormone.

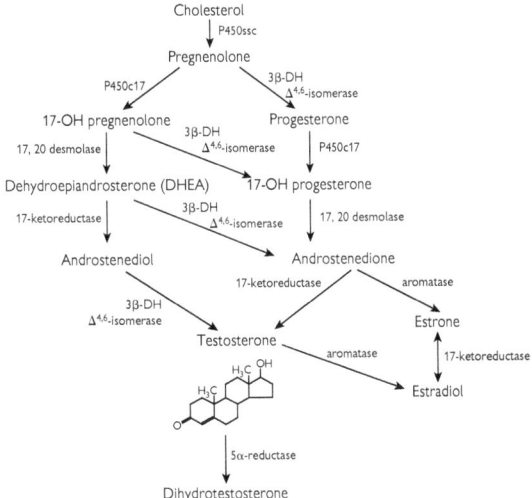

Figure 2.4 Gonadal steroid hormones.

Steroid-binding proteins

Because of their lipophilic properties, free steroid molecules are only sparingly soluble in water. In biological fluids, they are found either in a conjugated form, i.e., linked to a hydrophilic moiety (e.g., as sulfate or glucuronide derivatives), or bound to proteins (noncovalent, reversible binding).

In the plasma, unconjugated steroids are found mostly bound to carrier proteins. Binding to plasma albumin, accounting for 20–50% of the bound fraction, is rather unspecific, whereas binding to either corticosteroid-binding globulin (CBG) or the sex hormone–binding globulin (SHBG) is based on more stringent stereospecific criteria. The free fraction (1–10% of the total plasma concentration) is usually considered to represent the biologically active fraction.

Apart from the two functions mentioned above, the major roles of plasma-binding proteins appear to be (1) to act as a "buffer" or reservoir for active hormones and (2) to protect the hormone from peripheral metabolism (notably by liver enzymes) and increase the half-life of biologically active forms.

Further reading

Griffin JE, Ojeda SR, eds. (2004). *Textbook of Endocrine Physiology*, 5th ed. Oxford, UK: Oxford University Press.

Chapter 3

Menarche and adolescent gynecology

Introduction *24*
Hypothalamic–pituitary–gonadal axis *25*
Stages of puberty *27*
Precocious puberty *28*
Delayed puberty *29*
Further reading *30*

Introduction

Puberty marks the change from childhood to adolescence. In girls this means the development of breasts and secondary sexual hair and the onset of menstruation. At the same time, there is a period of accelerated growth. While the age at which the changes take place varies, it is abnormal for there to be no signs of secondary sexual development at the age of 14 years.

The trigger for the changes to start is an increasing frequency and amplitude of gonadotropin release. The ovaries are then stimulated to produce estrogen, which acts on the breast tissue to promote growth. This usually begins at around the age of 9 and takes about 5 years to be complete.

Pubic hair is stimulated by the release of androgens from the ovaries and the adrenal glands.

The age of menarche in girls appears to be decreasing, particularly in African-American girls. Factors such as general health, nutrition (weight), and exercise all seem to have a role in the age of onset.

Hypothalamic–pituitary–gonadal axis

During fetal life, GnRH activity from the hypothalamus (which is present from ~20 weeks) is suppressed by the steroid production from the fetoplacental unit. The ovaries thus have minimal estrogen output.

During infancy there is an increase in GnRH activity in boys aged 6 months and girls aged ~12 months. This leads to an increase in production of testosterone in boys and of estradiol in girls.

At this early age, the feedback mechanism to the pituitary is immature. As this feedback mechanism matures over a few months in childhood, the FSH and LH levels decrease. In girls, this leads to the lowest levels of FSH and LH at ~4 years old.

At ~6 years of age in girls, there is an increase in the amplitude and frequency of GnRH production from the hypothalamus. This is then associated with the onset of diurnal rhythms of FSH, LH, and steroids (see Fig. 3.1).

Puberty progresses with an increase in nocturnal amplitude of LH and a gradual change to the adult pattern of 90-minute pulses.

Boys

In boys, this diurnal rhythm results in peak testosterone in the early morning, leading to erections. Boys enter puberty ~6 months later than girls but are fertile earlier, with spermaturia from 6 mL of testicular volume.

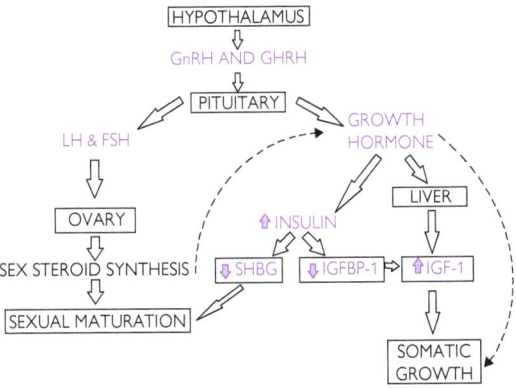

Figure 3.1 The origins, target organs, and feedback mechanisms providing the hypothalamic–pituitary–gonadal axis. FSH, follicle-stimulating hormone; GHRH, growth hormone–releasing hormone; GnRH, gonadotropin-releasing hormone; IGF-1, insulin-like growth factor 1; IGFBP-1, insulin-like growth factor binding protein 1; LH, luteinizing hormone; SHBG, sex hormone–binding globulin.

Girls
In girls, the diurnal rhythm results in a rise in estrogens later in the night, as it requires aromatization, thus giving peak values mid-morning. Subsequent ovulatory cycles develop 1–2 years after menarche.

FSH pulsatility shows no diurnal variation at any stage, with only a slight increase in amplitude, but not frequency, as puberty progresses.

Stages of puberty

In girls, breast and pubic hair development is described in five stages following the classification by Tanner (see Fig. 3.2).
- Sexual characteristics appear in 95% of girls between age 8.5 and 13 years.
- Breast development occurs between age 10 and 12.5 years (average age breast stage II = 11.2 years).
- Pubic hair usually occurs 6 months after breasts start, although before breasts in one-third of girls.
- 1 year later, there is an adolescent growth spurt.
- Menarche is at age 12–15 years, as growth spurt wanes; average age is 13 years.

Table 3.1 Tanner staging

Stage	Breast	Pubic hair
I	Preadolescent, elevation of papilla only	No pubic hair
II	Breast bud—elevation of breast papilla as small mound; enlargement of areolar diameter	Sparse growth of long, downy hair along labia
III	Further enlargement but no separation of contours	Hair coarser, darker, and more curled; over mons
IV	Projection of areola and papilla to form secondary mound above the level of breast	Adult-type hair but no spread to thigh
V	Mature, areola recessed to general contour of breast	Adult, with horizontal upper border and spread to thigh

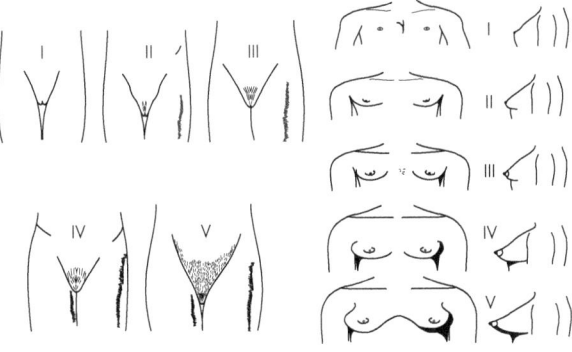

Figure 3.2 Tanner stages of puberty.

Precocious puberty

Precocious onset of puberty is defined as occurring younger than 2 standard deviations (SD) before the average age; <8 years old in females and <9 years in males. Its incidence is ~1 per 5000–10,000 individuals.

Causes of precocious puberty
- Idiopathic: family history and being overweight or obese accounts for 74% girls (60% boys). Transforming growth factor (TGF)-A may stimulate GnRH secretion.
- McCune–Albright syndrome (café-au-lait spots and polyostotic fibrous dysplasia)
- Tumors of the adrenal or ovary producing steroids, Peutz–Jeghers syndrome
- Cerebral tumors: intracranial lesions (tumors, hydrocephalus, CNS malformations, irradiation, trauma)—suspect tumor if patient is <3 years old.
- Ingestion of exogenous estrogens

The management of precocious puberty is initially to investigate and exclude tumors. A GnRH agonist (depot) can be used for suppression of the hypothalamic–pituitary–gonadal axis.

It is important to assess bone age (wrist) to predict potential epiphyseal fusion. These patients may benefit from receiving growth hormone, but this will depend on the age.

Delayed puberty

Delayed onset of puberty is defined as occurring older than 2 SD after the average age: >13.4 years old in females and >14 years in males.

A detailed history should be taken, with inquiries about general health. In girls, it is important to determine the age at which breast and pubic hair development started and if the girl had a growth spurt or still appears to be growing. Any chronic illness may lead to constitutional delay in puberty.

Examination should include accurate measurement of height and, in females, breast and pubic hair development. An internal examination should not be performed on girls.

Investigations
- Measurement of gonadotropins—FSH and LH—and estrogen
- Karotyping
- Ultrasound scan of the pelvis to confirm the presence of uterus and ovaries
- Possibly X-ray to determine bone age

Causes of delayed puberty

General
- Constitutional delay of growth and puberty. This is the most common condition seen by pediatric endocrinologists. It is usually associated with a positive family history, short stature, delayed epiphyseal maturation, and relatively short upper body. The height prognosis may be appropriate for parental centiles, although in severe cases the upper body may remain short. Treatment may be for psychological reasons, with very low-dose estrogen. Usually with the onset of breast development and a growth spurt the problem resolves.
- Malabsorption (e.g., celiac disease, inflammatory bowel disease)
- Underweight (dieting or anorexia nervosa, overexercise)
- Other chronic disease (malignancy, asthma, B-thalassemia major)

Gonadal failure (hypergonadotropic hypogonadism)
- Turner's syndrome (see Chapter 1)
- Postmalignancy (chemotherapy, local radiotherapy, or surgical removal)
- Polyglandular autoimmune syndromes

Gonadotropin deficiency
- Congenital hypogonadotropic hypogonadism (± anosmia). There are a number of possible diagnoses in this category:
- Idiopathic
- Kallmann's syndrome (X-linked)
  - Impaired migration of GnRH neurons
  - Anosmia, disturbance of color vision, dyskinesis

- Prader–Willi syndrome (autosomal dominant, chromosome 15): obesity, muscle hypotonia, mental retardation, short stature, small hands and feet, cryptorchidism
- Mutations in the pathway for GnRH secretion and action (KAL, DAX1, GnRH receptor, etc.).

These cases of hypogonadotropic hypogonadism may be difficult to distinguish from constitutional delay. Sometimes a GnRH test can be helpful, but results may be unreliable.
- Hypothalamic and pituitary lesions (tumors, post-radiotherapy); rare inactivating mutations of genes encoding LH, FSH, or their receptors

The management of delay in puberty will follow the diagnosis but is usually very low-dose estradiol (2 mcg slowly rising). A radical increase in estrogen will lead to abnormal breast development.

Further reading

Lissauer T, Clayden G (2007). *Illustrated Textbook of Paediatrics*, 3rd ed. London: Mosby Elsevier.

Chapter 4

Ovaries and the menstrual cycle

Introduction *32*
Hormones *34*
The ovary *36*
Follicular development *37*
Causes of anovulation and oligo-ovulation *38*

CHAPTER 4 Ovaries and the menstrual cycle

Introduction

Normally, ovulation occurs once a month in the fertile age range, between menarche and menopause, although anovulation generally occurs at the extremes of reproductive life. A cycle is regarded as normal if the duration is 24–35 days.

The time between menstruation and ovulation is termed the *follicular phase* and between ovulation and the next menstruation, the *luteal phase*.

Ovulation itself is the release of a mature, fertilizable oocyte from the dominant follicle, the culmination of an integrated, synchronized interplay of hormones from three principle sources:
- Anterior hypothalamus
  - Gonadotropin-releasing hormone (GnRH)
- Anterior pituitary
  - Follicle-stimulating hormone (FSH)
  - Luteinizing hormone (LH)
- Ovaries
  - 17-β estradiol
  - Progesterone

In addition, fine-tuning is provided by inhibin, activin, follistatin, and various growth factors.

Ovulation is achieved through the synchronization of the timing of release and quantity of the various hormones involved, which change throughout the cycle as a result of feedback mechanisms.

Fig. 4.1 is a very simple representation of the origin, target organ, and feedback mechanisms involving the hypothalamic–pituitary–ovarian axis. Fig. 4.2 is a diagrammatic representation of the important hormone levels at different stages in the cycle.

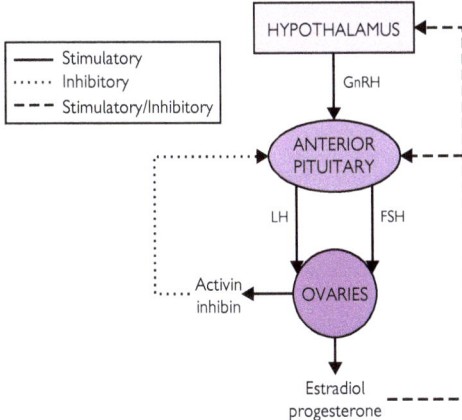

Figure 4.1 The origins, target organs, and feedback mechanisms involving the hypothalamic–pituitary–ovarian axis H, hypothalamus; P, pituitary; O, ovary; U, uterus.

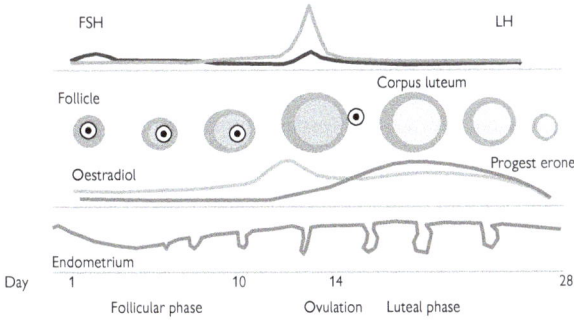

Figure 4.2 Hormone levels at various stages of the ovulatory cycle.

Hormones

Gonadotropin-releasing hormone (GnRH)
GnRH is secreted in a pulsatile fashion from nerve endings in the hypothalamus into the portal vessels running a short course to the anterior pituitary, where it induces the synthesis and release of FSH and LH. GnRH is undetectable in the peripheral circulation, but its pulsatile release, about once every hour, can be estimated from the LH pulses.

Both the frequency and amplitude of GnRH pulses vary greatly throughout the ovulatory cycle and are much less frequent but of greater amplitude in the luteal phase than in the follicular phase. The pattern of GnRH release is influenced by feedback mechanisms on the hypothalamus, which dictates the pattern of release of FSH and LH.

Follicle-stimulating hormone (FSH)
Immediately preceding menstruation, FSH levels start to rise as corpus luteum function fades, and they reach a peak around day 3 of menstruation. The FSH-stimulated growth of antral follicles, granulosa cell proliferation and differentiation, and aromatase action produce rising concentrations of estradiol and inhibin B, which exert a negative feedback mechanism. Other than a temporary increase at the time of the mid-cycle LH surge, FSH remains low until the end of the luteal phase.

FSH has several roles. It promotes the following:
- Granulosa cell proliferation and differentiation
- Antral follicle development
- Estrogen production
- Induction of LH receptors on the dominant follicle
- Inhibin synthesis

Luteinizing hormone (LH)
LH is the main promotor of the constant production of androgens, the substrate of ovarian steroid hormones, from theca cells. Concentrations of LH are uneventfully low throughout the ovulatory cycle, except for one tumultuous rise at mid-cycle to 10–20 times the resting levels. This surge lasts for 36–48 hours and is brought about by a dramatic effect of rapidly rising estradiol levels, which reach a certain concentration and initiate a switch from negative to positive feedback.

The preovulatory surge has several functions:
- Triggering of ovulation and follicular rupture
- Disruption of the cumulus–oocyte complex
- Induction of the resumption of oocyte meiotic maturation
- Luteinization of granulosa cells

Estradiol
17-β estradiol, the most important estrogen, is produced by granulosa cells under the influence of FSH, which promotes the action of the enzyme aromatase in converting basic androgens to estrogen.

The key functions of estradiol are as follows:
- Endometrial development
- Triggering of the LH surge at mid-cycle

- Suppression of FSH concentrations, thus aiding in the selection of the dominant follicle and preventing multifollicular development in the mid- to late follicular phase

Estradiol concentrations rise rapidly following menstruation to reach a peak in the late follicular phase and induce the LH surge. A slight decrease following ovulation is revived by production from the corpus luteum, until dropping sharply immediately before menstruation.

Progesterone

The main function of progesterone is to stimulate a secretory endometrium containing multiple differentiated glands receptive to a fertilized embryo, allowing it to implant. It also stimulates the expression of genes needed for implantation.

Because progesterone is produced by luteinized granulosa cells, its concentration only rises to significant amounts following ovulation and declines rapidly with the demise of the corpus luteum before menstruation. Progesterone reaches peak levels in the mid-luteal phase.

A blood sample for progesterone at this time, e.g., day 21 of a 28-day cycle or day 28 of a 35-day cycle, can be used to confirm ovulation; however, a single value is not predictive of the adequacy of the luteal phase.

The ovary

During the reproductive life span, the ovary is a dramatically changing organ. Fig. 4.3 is a diagrammatic representation of ovarian morphology. The inner, medullary or stromal, section is made up of connective tissue inundated with small capillaries and adrenergic nerves. The cortex contains an enormous number of oocyte-containing follicles ranging from ~300,000 at menarche to 1500 at menopause.

There is a constant state of flux in the various stages of development of the follicles, from primordial (an oocyte with a single layer of granulosa cells around it), through primary and secondary stages with increasing numbers of layers of granulosa cells, the antral stage containing follicular fluid, to a fully fledged, preovulatory follicle. A corpus luteum can be seen in the luteal phase of the cycle, and the picture is completed by the presence of corpora albicans (remnants of degenerate corpora lutea).

Although much of this changing picture of stages of follicular development is dependent on the stage of the (gonadotropin-dependent) ovulatory cycle, there is a constant, non-FSH-dependent, progression in development of primordial to potentially ovulatory follicles being available at the start of the ovulatory cycle, a process that may take ~10 weeks.

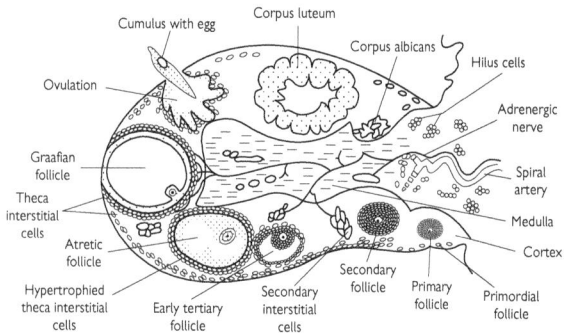

Figure 4.3 Diagrammatic representation of ovarian morphology.

Follicular development

One follicle a month (i.e., ~400 in a reproductive life span) will be selected to ovulate. The remainder, 99.9% of those that started life in the ovary, become atretic.

The earliest stage of follicular selection starts some 10 weeks before the cycle for which it is intended. This is a constant non-FSH-dependent step-up from primordial to several surviving, potentially ovulatory follicles 2–5 mm in diameter, which are made available. Sensitivity to FSH then comes into play to select the follicle for further growth, granulosa cell differentiation, and multiplication.

As estrogen and inhibin are produced by growing follicles, FSH concentrations are decreased, making it less available. The follicle most sensitive to FSH becomes dominant and the rest fade into atresia, starved of FSH.

The dominant follicle is the main producer of estradiol because of aromatase action stimulated by FSH. The dominant follicle also develops LH receptors in the late follicular phase in preparation for the LH surge and impending ovulation.

Causes of anovulation and oligo-ovulation

The causes of anovulation and oligo-ovulation (<9 ovulations in 1 year) are listed according to a modified World Health Organization (WHO) classification. The advantage of this type of classification is that it is treatment orientated—i.e., once the cause of the anovulation has been determined, the starting treatment for the induction of ovulation in that particular condition will be indicated.

The four groups of causes are as follows:
- Hypothalamic–pituitary failure (WHO Group I)
- Hypothalamic–pituitary dysfunction (WHO Group II)
- Ovarian failure (WHO Group III)
- Hyperprolactinemia (WHO Group IV)

Hypothalamic–pituitary failure

Otherwise known as hypogonadotropic hypogonadism, this is a condition in which gonadotropin concentrations are so low as to be unable to stimulate follicle development or ovarian steroidogenesis. Anovulation and amenorrhea are the consequences. There are several possible causes of this condition:
- Weight-related amenorrhea—the most common hypothalamic cause of anovulation, due to loss of weight as a result of severe dieting or frank anorexia nervosa
- Exercise-related amenorrhea—caused by very strenuous exercise such as marathon running and other athletic pursuits, and not uncommon in ballet dancers
- Stress-related—even moderate stress, e.g., moving, before examinations, long journeys involving time shifts, etc.
- Kallmann's syndrome—hypothalamic amenorrhea associated with anosmia (loss of the sense of smell).
- Debilitating diseases.
- Craniopharyngioma.
- Idiopathic—probably the most common cause of primary amenorrhea
- Surgical—hypophysectomy
- Radiotherapy for tumors of the pituitary or surrounding area
- Sheehan's syndrome—hypogonadotropic hypogonadism and hypopituitarism following severe postpartum hemorrhage

Hypothalamic–pituitary dysfunction

This dysfunction is characterized by normal FSH and estradiol concentrations, usually presenting as oligo- or amenorrhea. It comprises ~90% of all ovulatory disorders. In this group of ovulatory disorders, the vast majority are associated with polycystic ovary syndrome (PCOS).

About ~5% of all ovulatory disorders causing infertility are due to PCOS and are characterized by clinical and/or biochemical hyperandrogenism (hirsutism, persistent acne, raised testosterone concentrations) and a typical polycystic appearance of the ovary on ultrasound examination. Many women with PCOS are overweight or obese and hyperinsulinemic. The basic etiology is unknown, but it is thought to be associated with an overproduction of androgens by the ovaries which, in most of these women, seems to be genetic in origin. For a full description of this syndrome, see Chapter 5.

Ovarian failure

Ovarian failure is characterized by amenorrhea, hypoestrogenism, and high concentrations of FSH (often >25 IU/L). It is often accompanied at its onset by hot flashes. The ovaries in this condition are unable to respond to endogenous or exogenous FSH, as they are either completely devoid of oocytes or have a severely depleted reserve of oocytes.

Possible causes include the following:

- Onset of a "natural" menopause (>40 years of age).
- Premature menopause (<40 years of age)—which may be familial, related to fragile X promoter, or caused by a systemic autoimmune abnormality, chemotherapy, or direct radiation of the ovaries, but the underlying cause is often idiopathic
- Chromosomal abnormalities, e.g. Turner's syndrome (45, XO), characterized by typical physical features of short stature, cubitus valgus, webbed neck, and "streak" ovaries, and sometimes associated with aortic stenosis, presenting with primary amenorrhea.

Hyperprolactinemia

The presenting features of this cause of oligo- or anovulation are oligo/amenorrhea, infertility, and often, but not always, galactorrhea. Anovulation due to hyperprolactinemia is usually associated with serum prolactin concentrations, measured as an am fasting level, more than twice the upper limit of normal.

The major causes of hyperprolactinemia associated with anovulation are as follows:

- *Pituitary adenoma (prolactinoma)*—almost invariably benign tumors that secrete prolactin. According to their size, they may be termed macroadenomas (>10 mm in diameter) or microadenomas (<10 mm) when visualized by MRI or CT scan. When large, these adenomata may impinge on the optic chiasma, inducing a bitemporal hemianopia.
- *Hypothyroidism*. Thyroid-stimulating hormone (TSH) is released from the hypothalamus by TSH-releasing hormone, which is thought to be a prolactin-releasing hormone. Because TSH concentrations (and, by inference, those of TSH-releasing hormone) are often elevated in hypothyroid conditions, these may often be associated with hyperprolactinemia sufficient to cause anovulation.
- *Medications*—many drugs used in psychiatric conditions, as sedatives or antiemetics, suppress the hypothalamic secretion of dopamine. As dopamine is thought to be a prolactin-inhibiting factor, these medications can often induce hyperprolactinemia and a consequent anovulation. Oral contraceptives and other estrogen-containing medications may also induce a mild hyperprolactinemia, often associated with galactorrhea.

The treatment of these causes of anovulation is dealt with in Chapter 14.

Chapter 5

Polycystic ovary syndrome

Introduction 42
Definition 43
Prevalence 44
Etiology 44
Pathophysiology 45
Management 47
Long-term health implications of PCOS 50
Further reading 50

Introduction

In 1935, Stein and Leventhal first described the polycystic ovary as a frequent cause of irregular ovulation or anovulation in obese women seeking treatment for subfertility. The initial management of the condition was surgical, with wedge resection of the ovaries resulting in restoration of ovulation in the majority of cases.

In the last two decades, the polycystic ovary syndrome (PCOS) has been studied intensely, and although the exact etiology still escapes us, considerable knowledge of the prevalence, pathophysiology, and management of the syndrome has been gained.

Definition

The National Institutes of Health/National Institute of Child Health and Human Development (NIH/NICHD) (1990) definition of PCOS states that for a patient to be diagnosed with PCOS, she must have oligo-ovulation and hyperandrogenism (biochemical or clinical).

The European Society for Human Reproduction/American Society for Reproductive Medicine (ESHRE/ASRM) Rotterdam Consensus Meeting (2003)[1] proposed the following definition of PCOS, which has also been widely adopted.

Any two of the three are sufficient to confirm the diagnosis:
- Oligo- or anovulation
- Hyperandrogenism (biochemical or clinical)
- Polycystic ovaries on ultrasound examination

Syndromes with similar presenting features, e.g., congenital adrenal hyperplasia, androgen-secreting tumors, or Cushing's, should be excluded.

Oligo- or anovulation
Ovulation occurs at a frequency of less than once in 35 days.

Hyperandrogenism
Clinical signs of hyperandrogenism include hirsutism, acne, alopecia (male-pattern balding), and frank virilization. Biochemical indicators include raised concentrations of total testosterone and androstendione and elevated free androgen index.

Polycystic ovaries
This constitutes the presence in either ovary of ≥12 follicles measuring 2–9 mm in diameter and/or increased ovarian volume (>10 mL).

In practice, the diagnosis of PCOS can be made in almost every case without blood sampling. Although not essential for initial diagnosis or therapeutic decisions, for screening a blood sample for LH, total testosterone, FSH, fasting glucose, and fasting insulin may be taken. An oral glucose tolerance test is recommended for obese patients, especially for obese adolescents.

When suggested by the history of a rapid progress of hyperandrogenic symptoms, total testosterone concentration screens for androgen-producing tumors.

For 21-hydroxylase deficiency, serum 17-hydroxy-progesterone concentration is an excellent screening test.

If suspected, Cushing's syndrome can be detected using a 24-hour urinary cortisol or overnight dexamethasone suppression test.

---

1 Fauser B, Tarlatzis B, Chang J, Azziz R, et al. (2004). The Rotterdam ESHRE/ASRM-sponsored PCOS consensus workshop group. Revised 2003 consensus on diagnostic criteria and long-term health risks related to polycystic ovary syndrome (PCOS). *Hum Reprod* 19:41–47.

Prevalence

- PCOS is the most common female endocrinopathy, affecting 5–10% of women in their reproductive years.
- PCOS is associated with 75% of all anovulatory disorders causing infertility.
- Polycystic ovaries can be found in ~20% of the female population but are not necessarily associated with the typical symptoms.

Etiology

Uncertainty still surrounds the exact etiology of PCOS, although there is increasing evidence for genetic factors. The syndrome clusters in families, and prevalence rates in first-degree relatives are 5–6 times higher than in the general population.

About 70% of cases appear to be genetically transmitted. Intrauterine exposure of the female fetus to an excess of androgens is an etiological hypothesis finding increasing favor, although the source of the excess androgens is unknown.

The syndrome may also be acquired by an exposure to excess androgens at any time during the fertile time of life.

Pathophysiology

PCOS is a very heterogeneous syndrome in terms of both clinical presentation and laboratory manifestations. While the basic dysfunction seems to lie within the ovary, the clinical expression and severity of the symptoms are dependent on extraovarian factors, such as obesity, insulin resistance, and LH concentrations.

There are four main disturbances that may be involved in the pathophysiology of the syndrome:

- *Abnormal ovarian morphology:* ~6–8 times more preantral and small antral follicles are present in the polycystic ovary compared with the amount in the normal ovary. They arrest in development at a size of 2–9 mm, have a slow rate of atresia, and are sensitive to exogenous FSH stimulation. An enlarged stromal volume is invariably present, and a total ovarian volume >10 mL is often witnessed.
- *Excessive ovarian androgen production* lies at the heart of the syndrome. Almost every enzymatic action within the polycystic ovary that encourages androgen production is accelerated. Both insulin and LH, alone and in combination, exacerbate androgen production (Fig. 5.1).
- *Hyperinsulinemia* due to insulin resistance occurs in ~80% of women with PCOS and central obesity, but also in ~30–40% of lean women with PCOS. This is thought to be due to a postreceptor defect affecting glucose transport and is unique to women with PCOS. Insulin resistance, significantly exacerbated by obesity, is a key factor in the pathogenesis of anovulation and hyperandrogenism (Fig. 5.2).
- *Abnormality of pancreatic β-cell function* has also been described.

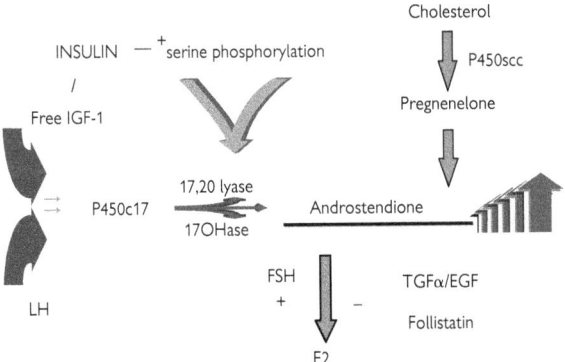

Figure 5.1 Mechanisms of excessive androgen production in the polycystic ovary. E2, estradiol; EGF, epidermal growth factor; FSH, follicle-stimulating hormone; LH, luteinizing hormone; TGFα, transforming growth factor α.

Excessive serum concentrations of LH are detected on single spot blood samples in ~40–50% of women with PCOS. High LH concentrations are more commonly found in lean than in obese women.

Although FSH serum concentrations are often within the low normal range, an intrinsic inhibition of FSH action may be present.

Prolactin concentrations may be slightly elevated.

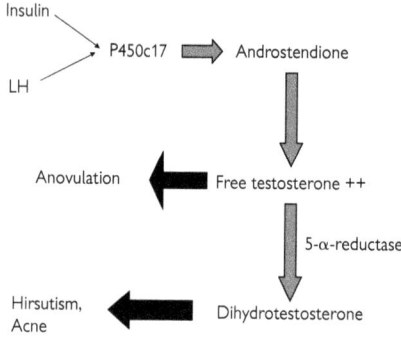

Figure 5.2 Insulin action as a key factor in the pathogenesis of anovulation and hyperandrogenism.

Management

The management of PCOS depends on the presenting symptoms. Whether these are symptoms of hyperandrogenism such as hirsutism and acne, oligo- or amenorrhea, or anovulatory infertility, the first-line treatment for the overweight or frankly obese patient must be loss of weight.

Weight loss

Obesity is a common feature in most women with PCOS. Increased truncal–abdominal fat in women with PCOS exacerbates insulin resistance and hyperandrogenism, and, consequently, the severity of the symptoms.

Fortunately, the reverse is also true, in that diet and exercise (lifestyle changes) are effective treatment. The loss of just 5% or more of body weight is capable of considerably reducing the severity of hirsutism and acne and restoring menstrual regularity and ovulation.

A motivation-inducing explanation of these facts should be given at the first consultation.

Hirsutism and acne

As many as 92% of women with hirsutism and 84% with persistent acne have PCOS as the underlying cause. A full description of management can be found in Chapter 6.

The first step for those who are overweight should be lifestyle changes to induce loss of weight. In most women, a loss of 5–10% of body weight is enough to greatly improve hirsutism within 6 months of weight reduction.

The combination of an antiandrogen, e.g., spironolactone (50–200 mg/day), and ethinylestradiol (EE, 35 micrograms/day) (co-cyprindiol) is very effective treatment when given cyclically. A significant improvement of acne can be achieved after 3 months and of hirsutism after 9 months of treatment.

Combined oral contraceptives (OCs) will also slowly improve hirsutism and acne but are less effective than specific antiandrogen medications.

Other antiandrogen medications used include flutamide and finasteride. Contraception is needed during their use.

Mechanical means of hair removal and more traditional treatment for persistent acne may also be used, especially when waiting for the medication to take effect.

Metformin, a well-established antidiabetic agent, is capable of reducing the degree of hirsutism and is recommended as first-line treatment when insulin resistance is diagnosed.

Anovulation and infertility

Weight loss should be the first-line treatment for overweight women desiring pregnancy. A reduction of 5% or more of body weight is often enough to restore ovulation and induce pregnancy and is also important for reducing miscarriage rates.

Clomifene citrate (CC) is the first-line medication for induction of ovulation. Given in a dose of 50–200mg/day from days 3 to 7 or from days 5 to 9 of a spontaneous or progestin-induced menstruation, clomifene will restore ovulation in ~75% and induce pregnancy in ~35–40%.

Failure to induce ovulation is more common in very obese patients and in those with very high serum androgen, insulin, or LH concentrations. Failure to respond to 300 mg/day, an endometrial thickness of <7 mm at mid-cycle, or failure to conceive following six ovulatory cycles requires a change in treatment mode. (For a detailed account, see Chapter 14.)

Metformin, a well-established oral antidiabetic agent, is capable of increasing ovulatory frequency in women with PCOS, apparently by decreasing insulin and androgen concentrations, in a dose of 1500–2500 mg/day (unlicensed). Its efficacy does not seem to depend on the presence of demonstrable insulin resistance, there is no evidence of teratogenicity, and it does not induce hypoglycemia in women with euglycemia.

Although clomifene is more efficient at inducing ovulation and pregnancy as first-line treatment as a mono-agent, metformin in combination with clomifene or added to clomifene for women who have proved clomifene resistance is a worthwhile strategy before proceeding to gonadotropin treatment. Gastrointestinal side effects are not uncommon.

Low-dose gonadotrophin therapy is designed to induce ovulation and conception while minimizing the complications due to multifollicular development, ovarian hyperstimulation syndrome (OHSS), and multiple pregnancies. Using a starting dose of 50–75 IU/day of FSH or human menopausal gonadotrophin (hMG) without a change of dose for the first 7–14 days and only small incremental dose rises of 25–37.5 IU for a minimum of 7 days where necessary, pregnancy rates of >20% per cycle may be expected.

Human chorionic gonadotropin (hCG) should be withheld if >3 follicles of diameter >16 mm are induced.

Fuller details can be found in Chapter 14.

Laparoscopic ovarian drilling (LOD) using cautery or laser has proved effective in restoring ovulation and inducing pregnancy, particularly in women of normal weight and with high concentrations of LH. Multiple pregnancy rate is low.

Some centers employ LOD when clomifene resistance is apparent. The morbidity of the surgical procedure must be considered when choosing this option.

In vitro fertilization (IVF) can be successfully employed for anovulatory women with PCOS when a further infertility-causing factor is involved or when the above methods of ovulation induction have been unsuccessful.

A suggested algorithm for the induction of ovulation for women with PCOS is shown in Fig. 5.3.

For a more detailed account of these methods of ovulation induction, see Chapter 14.

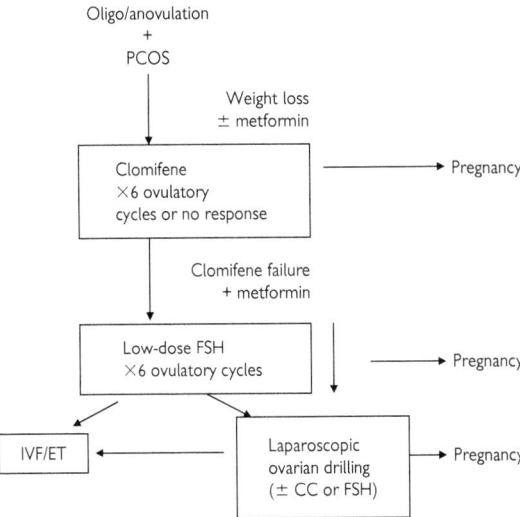

Figure 5.3 A suggested algorithm for the induction of ovulation for women with PCOS. Although less efficient than clomifene as first-line treatment, metformin is also capable of inducing ovulation. Laparoscopic ovarian drilling may be applied at any stage after clomifene resistance is evident. CC, clomifene citrate; ET, embryo transfer; FSH, follicle-stimulating hormone; IVF, in vitro fertilization.

Long-term health implications of PCOS

Women with PCOS who are obese, hyperinsulinemic, and hyperandrogenic are at substantial risk for the development of metabolic syndrome (syndrome X). If they remain untreated, the risk of developing diabetes mellitus is 7 times greater and of developing hypertension 4 times greater than in the general population.

Both of these conditions, as well as dyslipidemia and hyperhomocysteinemia, also common in PCOS, increase the risk of cardio- and cerebrovascular disease. Weight loss, diet, and exercise can reduce these dangers.

Women with PCOS have an increased incidence of gestational diabetes and of pregnancy-induced hypertension.

Endometrial cancer has a 5-fold increased incidence in PCOS due to unopposed estrogen action on the endometrium. This may be prevented by treating with a progestin-containing medication used cyclically or once every 3 months to induce uterine bleeding.

Endometrial hyperplasia may be treated similarly.

Further reading

Balen A, Conway GS, Homburg R, Legro R (2005). *Polycystic Ovary Syndrome—A Guide to Clinical Management*. London and New York: Taylor & Francis.

Chapter 6

Hirsutism and virilization

Introduction *52*
Pathophysiology *53*
History and examination *54*
Etiology *55*
Differential diagnosis *56*
Treatment *58*

Introduction

Hirsutism in the female is an excess of pigmented, thick terminal hair that appears in a male distribution in androgen-sensitive areas. These areas include face, chest, abdomen, and thighs. An excess of androgens will produce such hair growth in a male distribution.

Virilization is a much more progressive and serious form of hyperandrogenism and may include, in addition to hirsutism, male-pattern baldness, cliteromegaly, muscle development, and deepening of the voice.

Hirsutism may be due to hyperandrogenism from ovarian, adrenal, or iatrogenic (drug) sources. If not associated with irregular menstruation, it is probably familial, without underlying pathology.

Ethnic differences exist in the symptom of hirsutism, e.g., Mediterranean and Indian ethnicities may typically have more facial and body hair than do South and East Asians and Northern Europeans.

Pathophysiology

Androgens stimulate the development of the pilosebaceous unit, a common skin structure that gives rise to both hair follicles and sebaceous glands, found throughout the body except on the palms, soles, and lips.

Before puberty, body hair is primarily composed of fine, short, unpigmented vellous hairs that during pubarche are stimulated by androgens to become coarse, pigmented, thickened terminal hairs.

Following puberty in the female, excessive exposure to androgens may cause hirsutism by overstimulation of the transformation of fine, unpigmented vellous hairs to coarse, pigmented, thickened terminal hairs in skin areas sensitive to the effects of androgens. However, paradoxically, scalp hair responds to severe prolonged hyperandrogenism by loss of hair.

The hair growth cycle consists of three phases: active growth, resting phase, and shedding. The length of this cycle varies from 4 months on the face to 3 years on the scalp. This is important to know when assessing the response to treatment.

Androgens

Androgens are the main regulators of terminal hair growth. Testosterone is a strong androgen that binds to intracellular androgen receptors in the skin and is converted by 5α-reductase to dihydrotestosterone (DHT), which has even more potent androgen effects on the hair follicle and sebaceous gland. The concentration of free, biologically active testosterone, a crucial factor, is 2%.

Testosterone is bound by sex hormone–binding globulin (SHBG) (65%) and albumin (33%). Testosterone itself, obesity, and insulin lower SHBG concentrations, inducing increased activity of androgen action. The androgen receptor content will also influence the degree of androgen action on the hair follicle.

Androgens are produced by ovaries and adrenal glands. The basic androgen is androstendione, produced by both ovaries and adrenals; this is converted to testosterone, the major androgen, in both these organs.

At the level of the skin, testosterone is converted by 5α-reductase to DHT, which has a potent effect on the pilosebaceous unit. Dehydroepiandosterone and its sulfate (DHEAS) are produced mainly by the adrenals.

Ovarian androgens originate from theca cells, and their production is regulated by LH and insulin. Adrenal androgen production is regulated by ACTH.

Hyperandrogenism from ovarian, adrenal, or iatrogenic sources may produce symptoms of hirsutism, acne, alopecia, or virilism, depending on its degree.

History and examination

The rapidity of the onset and progression of hirsutism is a vital diagnostic indicator.

A rapid progression of symptoms, especially when accompanied by virilization, may be indicative of an ovarian or adrenal tumor.

A more insidious onset and progression of symptoms in the late teens, when accompanied by oligo- or amenorrhea, is due to polycystic ovary syndrome (PCOS) in ~90% of cases.

Hirsutism above the upper lip and on the limbs, especially when unaccompanied by menstrual disturbance or polycystic ovaries, is more likely to be familial. Enquiries or examination of other family members should be made.

On examination, in order to determine a baseline before initiating treatment, a full description of the location and severity of the hirsutism is required. This often suffices clinically, but a more specific estimation may be performed using a modified Ferriman–Gallwey score (Fig. 6.1).

Other signs of hyperandrogenism and virilization should be sought, i.e., acne, male-pattern balding or frank alopecia, or enlarged clitoris. Acanthosis nigricans, dark staining of the skin in the axillary or neck regions, indicates insulin resistance and is associated with obesity and PCOS.

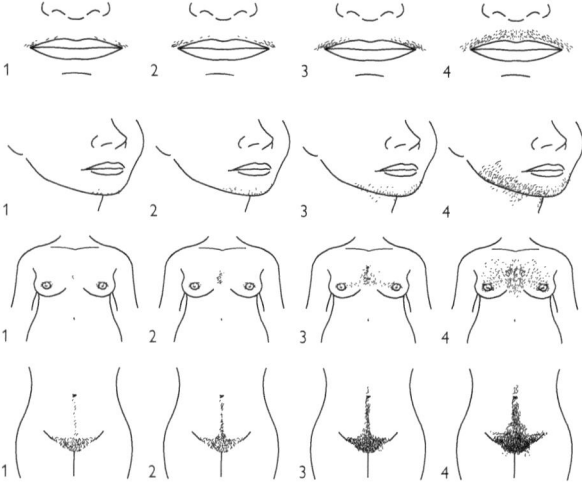

Figure 6.1 Modified Ferriman–Gallowey scale of hirsutism.

Etiology

- Familial
- Ovarian
- PCOS
- Androgen-producing tumors
- Adrenal
- Congenital adrenal hyperplasia (CAH)
- Cushing's syndrome
- Neoplasms
- Iatrogenic
- Anabolic steroids
- Danazol
- Phenytoin

Differential diagnosis

Familial
This form usually presents as excessive hair growth on the forearms, lower limbs, and upper lip, which is often evident in close family members. Ovarian function is normal and periods are regular, as are androgen concentrations.

Familial hirsutism is both typical and natural in certain populations, such as in some women of Mediterranean ancestry.

PCOS
An insidious onset of hirsutism accompanied by oligo- or amenorrhea is enough to make the diagnosis of PCOS. In a large majority of cases, this may be confirmed by an ultrasonic vaginal examination of the ovaries demonstrating >12 follicles between 2 and 9 mm in diameter and/or an ovarian volume >10 mL.

Obesity, which often accompanies PCOS, exaggerates the symptoms of hyperandrogenism.

Hormonal manifestations are not required for the diagnosis, but raised serum testosterone concentrations are often found. Concentrations of LH are frequently high, especially in women with PCOS of normal weight, and insulin resistance, detected by a fasting glucose:insulin ratio of <4.5, on a glucose tolerance test or by more sophisticated methods, is very prevalent, especially in overweight and frankly obese patients.

See Chapter 5 on PCOS for more details.

Androgen-producing tumors
The hallmark of these fortunately rare tumors is a rapid onset and progression of symptoms. Hirsutism may be rapidly followed by symptoms and signs of virilization. Testosterone levels are extremely high, often in the male range, with ovarian androgen-producing tumors, and DHEAS levels are very high with adrenal tumors.

Ultrasound of ovaries and MRI or CT scans of ovaries are required to confirm the diagnosis.

Ovarian and adrenal vain sampling is required to localize a tumor.

Congenital adrenal hyperplasia (CAH)
CAH is a partial block of enzyme action in the cascade involved in eventual cortisol synthesis in the adrenal. The partial block induces an increased discharge of ACTH and a consequent accumulation of androgens.

The most common form is 21-hydroxylase deficiency, which is particularly prevalent in Hispanics and Ashkenazi Jews. Almost invariably, the CAH seen by gynecologists is a mild form of 21-hydroxylase deficiency with an onset of hyperandrogenic symptoms in early adult life (late onset, LOCAH). Very high serum concentrations of 17-hydroxyprogesterone, 10–400 times higher than normal values, establish the diagnosis.

Rarer forms of LOCAH, 11β-hydroxylase and 3β-hydroxysteroid dehydrogenase deficiencies, require dynamic testing with ACTH for accurate diagnosis.

PCOS is almost invariably found in association with CAH.

Other possible diagnoses

Luteoma of pregnancy driven by hCG can produce symptoms of hyperandrogenism. They may be diagnosed in the early stages of pregnancy by ultrasound examination, need no treatment, and regress spontaneously following delivery.

Cushing's syndrome may cause hirsutism but has other very characteristic features that do not usually present to the gynecologist.

The key laboratory investigations are total testosterone, which will be very high (often in the male range) in the case of ovarian androgen-producing tumors, as is DHEAS in adrenal tumors. These diagnoses must be ruled out, especially in the presence of rapidly progressive symptoms.

In certain populations, 21-hydroxylase-deficient LOCAH is prevalent and can be excluded by measuring a basal morning serum 17-hydroxyprogesterone concentration (cutoff value, 20 nmol/L) in the proliferative phase.

Treatment

When hirsutism is accompanied by overweight or frank obesity, as is often the case in PCOS, weight loss should be the first line of treatment. For obese women with PCOS, a loss of 5–10% of body weight is enough to improve hirsutism greatly in 40–55% of women within 6 months of weight reduction. Weight loss has the undoubted advantages of being effective and cheap with no side effects.

Metformin, a well-established oral antidiabetic agent, is capable of reducing insulin and androgen concentrations in women with PCOS. Although it may have a therapeutic effect on the degree of hirsutism, it cannot be recommended as the first-line treatment when hirsutism is the main presenting symptom.

Mechanical means of hair removal may be used as a short-term solution to hirsutism or as an adjuvant to medical treatment, especially when waiting for the medication to take effect.

Surgical removal is required for all androgen-producing tumors.

When LOCAH is the established cause of hirsutism, the administration of dexamethasone, 0.5 mg at bedtime, is capable of completely reversing the symptoms. Given the length of the hair growth cycle, this will take 3–9 months to start the improvement, but no other medication is required.

Combined oral contraceptives (COCs) that do not contain androgenic progestogen will slowly improve hirsutism by suppressing LH and increasing SHBG concentrations. However, antiandrogenic medications are a more specific and more effective treatment for hirsutism.

A number of antiandrogen medicines that block the synthesis or action of androgens may be used for the treatment of hirsutism: spironolactone, flutamide, and finasteride. They must be used in conjunction with a contraceptive agent.

Spironolactone

Spironolactone is an aldosterone antagonist whose antiandrogen action is exerted by competitive inhibition of testosterone and DHT binding to the androgen receptor. In the usual dose of 100 mg/day, spironolactone may induce some menstrual disturbances, particularly polymenorrhea, which is often transient and resolves within a few months. Mild breast tenderness occurs frequently.

Spironolactone has been widely used for the treatment of hirsutism. A 40% reduction of the hirsutism score after 6 months may be expected, similar to that obtained with flutamide and finasteride.

Flutamide

Flutamide is a nonsteroidal antiandrogen that has been used primarily in advanced prostatic carcinoma, in that it inhibits DHT binding to the androgen receptors. It has also proved effective in the treatment of hirsutism and acne in women. Similar improvements of hirsutism have been reported whether doses of 250 or 500 mg/day are used.

The efficacy, noninterference with ovulation, and generally good tolerance of flutamide have been tempered by rare reports of hepatotoxicity, which may be severe; its incidence seems to increase with higher doses.

Careful monitoring of liver function is therefore advised if flutamide is to be used for the treatment of hirsutism.

Finasteride

Finasteride acts by inhibiting the activity of 5α-reductase, the enzyme responsible for the conversion of testosterone to DHT, which is particularly potent at the hair follicle level. Taken orally in a dose of 1–5 mg/day, it is effective without any appreciable side effects, although it may need prolonged treatment to achieve the goal.

Finasteride is thought to be effective in the treatment of hirsutism regardless of the cause, as 5α-reductase has a vital role in the androgen regulation of hair growth, and its inhibition is thus potentially effective. As with spironolactone and flutamide, contraceptive use is recommended with finasteride, to avoid the potential risk of feminization of a male fetus.

However effective these antiandrogen medicines may be, they ameliorate symptoms while they are being taken but fail to cure the cause. After withdrawal of treatment with spironolactone, flutamide, or finasteride, hirsutism relapses to 60–80% of the original score.

An essential element in successful compliance of the patient on antiandrogen treatment is the accuracy and fullness of information given to her. She should be told first and foremost that a good clinical response to treatment takes time; second, of the need for long-term maintenance treatment of 3–4 years, even when obvious clinical improvement has been achieved; and third, of the possibility of relapse some time after treatment is terminated.

Chapter 7

Amenorrhea and oligomenorrhea

Introduction *62*
Etiology *63*
Investigations *67*
Management *70*

Introduction

Amenorrhea is the absence of menstruation for at least 6 months. *Primary amenorrhea* is defined as a menstrual period never occurring, and *secondary amenorrhea* is absence of menstruation after at least one period.

Oligomenorrhea is the occurrence of menstruation less than once in 35 days to 6 months or <9 times in 1 year.

Etiology

Physiological amenorrhea is an acceptable diagnosis:
- Before the onset of menarche, unless this has not occurred before the age of 17 years
- Following menopause, if this occurs after the age of 40 years
- During pregnancy
- During lactation

All other causes of amenorrhea and oligomenorrhea are listed according to a modified World Health Organization (WHO) classification. The five groups of causes are as follows:
- Hypothalamic–pituitary failure (WHO Group I)
- Hypothalamic–pituitary dysfunction (WHO Group II)
- Ovarian failure (WHO Group III)
- Hyperprolactinemia (WHO Group IV)
- Outflow tract defect (WHO Group V)

The classification of oligo- and amenorrhea, their common causes, and hormonal profiles are summarized in Table 7.1.

Hypothalamic–pituitary failure

Amenorrhea in this condition is due to hypogonadotropic hypogonadism, in which concentrations of both FSH and LH are so low as to be unable to stimulate follicle development or ovarian steroidogenesis. Amenorrhea, anovulation, and hypoestrogenism are the consequences. There are several possible causes of this condition:
- Weight-related amenorrhea—a common cause of amenorrhea, due to loss of weight during severe dieting or frank anorexia nervosa
- Exercise-related amenorrhea—caused by very strenuous exercise such as marathon running and other athletic pursuits, and common in ballet dancers
- Stress related—even moderate stress, e.g., moving, before examinations, long trips involving time zone shifts
- Kallmann's syndrome—hypothalamic amenorrhea associated with anosmia (loss of the sense of smell)
- Debilitating systemic diseases
- Craniopharyngioma
- Idiopathic—probably the most common cause of primary amenorrhea
- Surgical—hypophysectomy
- Radiotherapy for tumors of the pituitary or surrounding area
- Sheehan's syndrome—hypogonadotropic hypogonadism and hypopituitarism following severe postpartum hemorrhage

Hypothalamic–pituitary dysfunction

WHO Group II may present as oligo- or amenorrhea and comprises the vast majority of these disorders. Characterized by normal FSH and estradiol concentrations, almost all cases are associated with polycystic ovary syndrome (PCOS) (see Chapter 5).

Briefly, PCOS is characterized by oligo- or amenorrhea, clinical and/or biochemical hyperandrogenism (hirsutism, persistent acne, raised

CHAPTER 7 Amenorrhea and oligomenorrhea

Table 7.1 Classification of oligo- and amenorrhea, common causes, and hormonal profiles

WHO Group	Name	Common causes	Hormonal profile
I	Hypothalamic–pituitary failure Hypogonadotropic Hypogonadism	Weight, exercise, stress related Kallmann's syndrome Sheehan's syndrome Hypophysectomy, radiotherapy Tumors Idiopathic	Very low FSH, LH, E2
II	Hypothalamic–pituitary dysfunction	PCOS CAH	Low or normal FSH High or normal LH High or normal testosterone
		Cushing's syndrome Androgen-producing tumors	High 17-OH prog. High cortisol Very high testosterone
III	Ovarian failure	Autoimmune Infections Surgery, irradiation Gonadal dysgenesis Idiopathic, familial	High FSH, LH (LH may be normal in early stages). Low E2
IV	Hyperprolactinemia	Pituitary adenoma Medication Stress Hypothyroidism	High prolactin Low FSH, LH High TSH
V	Outflow tract defect	Imperforate hymen Transverse vaginal septum Asherman's syndrome Absent uterus Cervical stenosis Androgen insensitivity Hermaphroditism	Normal Testosterone—male

testosterone concentrations), and a typical polycystic appearance of the ovary on ultrasound examination. Two or more of these three diagnostic points are enough to confirm the diagnosis, assuming other causes of hyperandrogenism have been ruled out.

Many women with PCOS are overweight or obese, hyperinsulinemic, and infertile. The basic etiology is unknown, but it is thought to be associated with an overproduction of androgens by the ovaries. In most of these women, this overproduction appears to be genetic in origin.

Ovarian failure

Ovarian failure is responsible for ~10% of women diagnosed with secondary amenorrhea before the age of 40 years (premature menopause), but it may also be a cause of primary amenorrhea. This form of amenorrhea is characterized by hypoestrogenism and high concentrations of FSH (often >25 IU/L).

The ovaries in this condition are unable to respond to endogenous or exogenous FSH, as they are either completely devoid of oocytes or have a severely depleted reserve of oocytes. Possible causes follow.

Secondary amenorrhea—premature menopause
- Familial or genetic (e.g., fragile X permutation)
- Autoimmune abnormality
- Iatrogenic—chemotherapy or direct radiation of the ovaries, pelvic surgery
- Debilitating systemic disease
- Infectious, e.g., mumps
- Idiopathic.

Primary amenorrhea
- Chromosomal abnormalities—gonadal dysgenesis, e.g., Turner's syndrome (45, XO), characterized by typical physical features of short stature, cubitus valgus, webbed neck, and "streak" ovaries, and sometimes associated with aortic stenosis
- Intersexuality and hermaphroditism

Hyperprolactinemia

Hyperprolactinemia may be a cause of either oligo- or amenorrhea, infertility, and often, but not always, galactorrhea. (Conversely, galactorrhea is not always accompanied by hyperprolactinemia.)

Common causes of hyperprolactinemia include the following:
- *Pituitary adenoma* (prolactinoma)—almost invariably benign tumors that secrete prolactin. According to their size, they may be termed *macroadenomas* (>10 mm in diameter) or *microadenomas* (<10 mm) when visualized by MRI or CT scan. When large, these adenomata may impinge on the optic chiasma, inducing a bitemporal hemianopia.
- *Hypothyroidism*. Thyroid-stimulating hormone (TSH)-releasing hormone is also thought to be a prolactin-releasing hormone. As TSH concentrations (and, by inference, TSH-releasing hormone) are often elevated in hypothyroid conditions, these may often be associated with hyperprolactinemia sufficient to cause oligo- or amenorrhea.
- *Medications*—many drugs used in psychiatric conditions, as sedatives or antiemetics, suppress the hypothalamic secretion of dopamine. Because dopamine is thought to be a prolactin-inhibiting factor, these medications can often induce hyperprolactinemia and a consequent oligo- or amenorrhea. Oral contraceptives and other estrogen-containing medications may also induce a mild hyperprolactinemia, often associated with galactorrhea.
- *Stress*, particularly if prolonged, may cause a hyperprolactinemia sufficient to induce oligo- or amenorrhea.

Outflow tract defects

Unlike the causes of amenorrhea, outflow tract defects are not usually associated with anovulation but with a mechanical defect preventing menstruation. Possible causes include the following:
- Imperforate hymen
- Congenital absence of the uterus (see Chapter 1)
- Transverse vaginal septum
- Severe intrauterine adhesions, endometrial damage (Asherman's syndrome)
- Cervical stenosis

Investigations

The importance of a detailed gynecological and medical history cannot be emphasized enough. By listening carefully to the patient and asking the correct direct questions, followed by a thorough gynecological and general physical examination, the clues obtained will often point toward the diagnosis and dictate the order in which examinations should be performed. Using this approach and good common sense, laboratory examinations, expense, and time can be limited to a minimum.

A suggested checklist is presented in Table 7.2.

A rapid scheme for the diagnosis of amenorrhea is shown as a flowchart in Fig. 7.1. Minimal laboratory examinations are required in this scheme, as endogenous estrogen production can be estimated by a progestin withdrawal test for amenorrhea. This is unnecessary if oligo- and not amenorrhea is the presenting complaint.

This leaves only prolactin to be measured. For a negative progestin withdrawal, FSH concentrations are measured to see if the problem is hypogonadotropic or hypergonadotropic hypogonadism.

An outflow tract defect can be diagnosed if both progestin and estrogen/progestin withdrawal do not produce bleeding and FSH levels are in the normal range.

Table 7.2 Checklist for history-taking and physical examination of the amenorrheic patient

History

Age—female partner
Occupation
Previous pregnancies
Duration of amenorrhea—primary or secondary
Previous regularity of menstruation
Past medical and surgical history
Intercurrent illnesses, medications, drugs, alcohol use
Family history
Previous contraception
Age at menarche
Sexual activity and problems
Direct questions, where relevant:
   Sense of smell? Abdominal pain? Physical activity?
   Serious changes in weight or diet?
   Hot flashes? Hirsutism, acne, or galactorrhea?

Examination

Body build
Weight, height, body mass index
General physical examination
Distribution of hair growth, hirsutism
Breasts, galactorrhea
Acne
Gynecological examination
   Vulva, vagina, cervix, uterus, adnexae

CHAPTER 7 **Amenorrhea and oligomenorrhea**

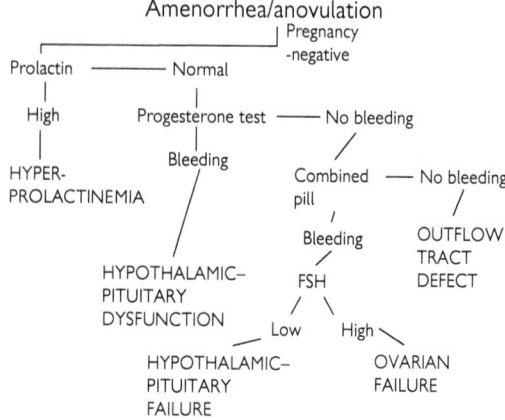

Figure 7.1 A rapid scheme for the diagnosis of amenorrhea and anovulation.

Once the type of amenorrhea has been classified in this way, a secondary round of investigation may be initiated, e.g.:
- Hypothalamic–pituitary failure—test for anosmia, systemic diseases, secondary sex characteristics, weight loss
- Hypothalamic–pituitary dysfunction—this group is further examined as for oligomenorrheic patients (see Fig. 7.2).
- Ovarian failure—karyotype, autoimmune antibodies
- Fragile X
- Hyperprolactinemia—TSH, MRI of pituitary region
- Outflow tract defect—pelvic ultrasound examination, karyotype if uterus is absent

If oligomenorrhea is the presenting symptom, the scheme illustrated in Fig. 7.2 will be helpful.

In any of these situations, the aim is to arrive at a correct diagnosis for the cause of the oligo- or amenorrhea in the minimum amount of time and with a minimum of investigations. As this classification is very much treatment orientated, once the diagnosis is made, it will help in determining the correct treatment that is suitable for that specific diagnosis.

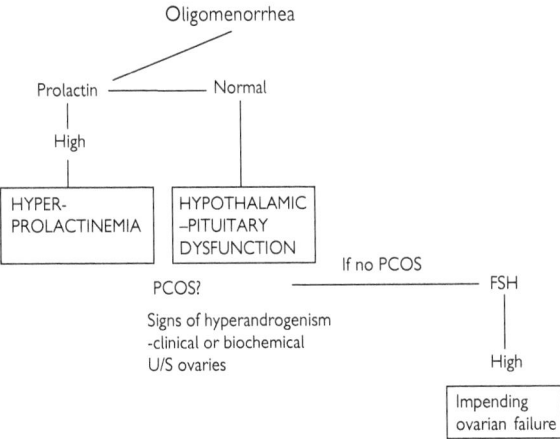

Figure 7.2 Investigations of oligomenorrhea.

Management

The treatment of oligomenorrhea and amenorrhea depends not only on the etiology but also on the purpose of the treatment—basically whether there is a problem of infertility or not. Except for women with outflow tract defect, the rest of the patients may be assumed to have oligo- or anovulation and, if pregnancy is desired, ovulation induction will be needed. This is dealt with thoroughly in Chapter 14 and is mentioned only briefly in the following list of possible treatment modes.

Hypothalamic–pituitary failure

For ovulation induction, gonadotropin treatment, which must contain both FSH and LH, is very effective. If the pituitary is intact, pulsatile GnRH therapy is equally effective. If the cause of the amenorrhea is low body weight, it is highly recommended that the patient gain weight before embarking on ovulation induction therapy in order to avoid associated complications of pregnancy.

If pregnancy is not wanted, hormone replacement therapy (HRT) with estrogens and progesterone, similar to that used in menopause, is called for to avoid osteoporosis or any other possible effects of prolonged hypoestrogenism.

Referral to reproductive endocrinologist is recommended.

Hypothalamic–pituitary dysfunction

For women diagnosed as having PCOS and suffering infertility, the full range of possible treatments for ovulation induction is described in Chapter 5. These include weight loss, clomifene citrate, metformin and other insulin sensitizers, and low-dose gonadotropin therapy.

For those who have PCOS but for whom infertility is not the presenting complaint, several options are open and may be tailored to the individual case.

Weight loss is an essential first step for overweight or frankly obese patients. A loss of just 5% or more of body weight may be enough to restore ovulation and menstruation.

For those suffering from symptoms of hyperandrogenism (hirsutism, acne, alopecia), a combination of an antiandrogen spironolactone and oral contraceptive is probably the most widely used treatment. Oral contraceptives have an antiandrogen action at several sites: (1) suppression of LH release by the anterior pituitary; (2) suppression of the action of 5-reductase; and (3) increase in SHBG concentrations.

The combination of spironolactone (100–200 mg) and an oral contraceptive given cyclically has proven to be very effective in the treatment of hirsutism and acne. It also helps restore regular menstruation and provides contraception. An impressive reduction in the degree of hirsutism can occur after 9 months of treatment, and acne has been successfully treated.

Patients need to be informed that this treatment is not instant and that at least 4–9 months are needed to see an improvement in hirsutism and 3–5 months for acne, whereas menstruation is restored following the first treatment cycle. Further details and those of other antiandrogen preparations can be found in Chapter 6.

Metformin, an oral insulin-lowering and antidiabetic agent, has also been found to be effective in restoring ovulation and regular menstruation in women with PCOS. It is given in a dose of 1500–2500 mg daily in divided daily doses. See Chapter 14 for further details.

Ovarian failure

For patients desiring pregnancy, ovum donation is the only successful option. Otherwise, HRT, as for menopausal patients, is recommended.

Hyperprolactinemia

When hyperprolactinemia and oligo- or amenorrhea are associated with medication, the benefits and disadvantages of reducing the dosage or withdrawing medication must be carefully weighed. Hypothyroidism as a cause should be treated with the appropriate medication for correction of thyroid function rather than with specific prolactin-lowering agents. All other cases of hyperprolactinemia associated with ovulatory dysfunction and oligo or amenorrhea, whether idiopathic or from a pituitary tumor, require treatment.

Neurosurgical treatment for hyperprolactinemia is very rarely required. For both micro- and macroprolactinomas, prolactin-lowering drugs are safer, more efficient, and often capable of causing tumor shrinkage without recourse to surgery.

Surgery should be reserved only for the very rare case completely resistant to medication, for nonsecreting pituitary adenomas or parasellar tumors, and in those who have severe visual disturbances that fail to improve with medication. For all the rest, prolactin-lowering medication will serve the purpose adequately.

Many dopamine agonists are in use for the treatment of infertility associated with hyperprolactinemia.

Bromocriptine

Bromocriptine is the most widely used dopamine agonist. Provided in tablets of 2.5 mg, it is wise to start with half a tablet at bedtime, taken with food, for the first week to 10 days of treatment. This tends to help avoid the rather unpleasant side effects of this drug, i.e., nausea, vomiting, diarrhea, and postural hypotension. Following this initial dosage regime, 2.5 mg nightly can be given, which may be titrated up to a maximum dose of even 20 mg/day, although this is rarely needed for restoration of ovulation and menstruation.

The best way of gauging the dose is restoration of regular menstruation. This is a better indicator than the serum prolactin concentration that the correct dose is being administered.

Follow-up of tumor size by MRI or CT is needed only when no response is seen, either by the return of regular ovulation or at least by a reduction in serum prolactin concentrations. Restoration of menstruation is achieved in ~85% of cases, even including those with a macroprolactinoma. This is a remarkably successful and simple treatment and has the additional advantage that it is capable of reducing the size of the prolactinomata and, often, with continued treatment, microprolactinomata will disappear altogether.

Cabergoline

Cabergoline is at least equally as effective as bromocriptine and has the added advantage that it is long acting. A single oral dose can lower prolactin concentrations for 1–2 weeks.

For the resumption of ovulatory cycles, the recommended dose is 0.5–2 mg/week, usually divided into a twice-weekly dosage.

Outflow tract defects

Imperforate hymen and transverse vaginal septa are treated with surgical techniques to restore the integrity of the outflow tract. Imperforate hymen is probably the most frequent obstructive anomaly of the female genital tract; estimates of its frequency vary from 1 case per 1000 population to 1 case per 10,000 population.

The diagnosis is sometimes made in infancy, with the infant noted to have a bulging, yellow-gray mass at or beyond the introitus. More commonly, it presents at puberty with cyclical pelvic and abdominal pain and amenorrhea. Treatment is via cruciate incision in the hymen.

A transverse septum is also excised surgically, but it can be large and the surgery can be complicated. Skin grafting may be required. This surgery is best referred to those with expertise and access to plastic surgery consultations.

Restoration of endometrial function, damaged by intrauterine adhesions or overzealous curettage, is more complicated and less successful. Operative hysteroscopy to remove adhesions is the most popular option. Insertion of an intrauterine contraceptive device for 3–6 months has also met with some success. Both of these treatment modes are usually supported by a course of antibiotics and estrogen.

Chapter 8

Menopause and hormone replacement therapy

Introduction 74
Pathophysiology 74
Other hormonal changes 75
Symptoms 75
Women's Health Initiative (WHI) trial 79
Risks and benefits of HRT 80
HRT preparations 81
Alternative treatment 82

Introduction

The term *menopause* is derived from the Greek *menos* (month) and *pauses* (cessation), but the term has come to be used to describe the climacteric, which again is derived form the Greek *klimakter* (rung of ladder).

The average age at which menopause occurs has not changed, but life expectancy has improved to the extent that in the United States, women can expect to spend about one-third of their lives in a menopausal state.

- *Menopause:* defined retrospectively 1 year after last menstrual period; average age 51
- *Climacteric:* the prodrome surrounding the transition to menopause; average age 45–47 (lasting 4 years on average—up to 10 years)
- *Premature ovarian failure:* <40 years

Pathophysiology

The number of primordial follicles that a female has shrinks throughout life, with there being no replacement.

- Newborn   2 million
- Puberty   300,000–400,000
- 40 years+   Few thousand
- Postmenopause   Few or no ova

The number of ovarian follicles available to mature each cycle is depleted (300–400 cycles on average) as women get older. As one oocyte ovulates, ~1000 become atretic through apoptosis.

There are two critical landmarks in the ovarian failure process: the first is a marked decline in fertility (no cycle dysfunction) and the second occurs when the menstrual cycle changes become noticeable, with a shortened follicular phase and luteal dysfunction.

The effect of the reduced pool of follicles for stimulation is that the estrogen levels start to fall. Initially there is a "compensated failure." This is then associated with an increase in the production of FSH and a decrease in the level of inhibin produced by the follicles.

Early follicular inhibin B and FSH appear to be predictive of ovarian reserve and of response to gonadotropin stimulation. The FSH level will, however, vary in the climacteric with a nonlinear increase; currently, more population data on inhibin B are awaited. Given the lack of more population data on inhibin B, the standard test remains FSH alone.

"Decompensated failure" occurs when the follicle pool is very low. FSH rises further (10- to 20-fold); LH rises 3-fold (shorter half-life). Estrogen levels drop due to reduction in follicle number and qualitative effect on granulosa cell aging. Progesterone production ceases; this can lead to endometrial proliferation and hyperplasia.

In the developed world, there is an increasing female life expectancy but unaltered age of menopause.

Other hormonal changes

Adrenal and ovarian androgens (testosterone and androstendione) decline. Some testosterone is still, however, produced by theca cells. Ovarian androstenedione production drops by half during menopause so that the majority is from the adrenals (1:4 ratio).

Sex hormone–binding globulin (SHBG) decreases from reduction in ovarian estradiol. The main postmenopausal estrogen is estrone. It is produced primarily in peripheral adipose tissue and postmenopausal ovary by aromatization of adrenal androstenedione. The amount of estrone produced is related to body weight and age. Glucocorticoid administration in postmenopausal women will suppress estrogen production, confirming that it is from an adrenal production site.

Insulin resistance rises after the menopause. This change results in an increase in central adiposity (android rather than gynecoid shape) and a decreased lean body mass.

Symptoms

The characteristic symptoms of the menopause are listed in Table 8.1.

Hot flashes

The hot flash, though it may characteristically start over the face or neck area, involves the whole body and is often followed by intense sweating and then shivering (see Fig. 8.1). Hot flashes occur in 70% of Caucasian and Afro-Caribbean women but are less common in Asians.

Hot flashes do not occur in women with Turner's syndrome or life-long hypothalamic amenorrhea, and obese women are partially protected, probably by their high estrone production and lower SHBG levels.

Table 8.1 Symptoms of menopause

Acute	Intermediate/late
Hot flashes (70%)	Dyspareunia
Night sweats (70%)	Loss of libido
Insomnia	Urethral syndrome
Anxiety/irritability	Vaginal atrophy
Memory loss	
Poor concentration	
Mood changes	

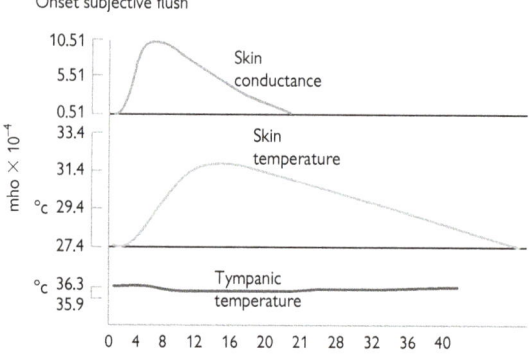

Figure 8.1 Physiology of the hot flash. Reprinted with permission from Tataryn IV, Lomax P, Bajorek JG, Chesarek W, Meldrum DR, Judd HL (1980). Postmenopausal hot flushes: a disorder of thermoregulation. *Maturitas* 2:101–107.

The mechanism is thought to involve estrogen's altering of hypothalamic opioid and serotonergic activity; the loss of this activity can lead to thermodysregulation, mediated by noradrenaline. Estrogen also increases α_2-adrenergic activity, hence the rationale for clonidine therapy.

CNS system

Estrogen and progesterone receptors are colocated in the central nervous system (CNS) in the hypothalamus, amygdala, preoptic area, hippocampus, and cerebellum. In these areas, they mediate genomic effects, e.g., limbic system functions subserving emotion and behavior.

Estrogen has a direct effect on 5-hydroxytryptamine (5-HT; serotonin) and noradrenaline receptors. It increases the rate of degradation of monoamine oxidase (MAO), thus increasing levels of 5-HT. Estrogen also displaces tryptophan from albumin, providing more 5-HT substrate as well as enhancing the transport of 5-HT.

The depression seen at menopause is partly due to a serotonin and noradrenaline deficit. Estrogen increases the levels of these neurotransmitters. The effect of estrogen supplementation in the form of HRT during menopause on cognitive function is unclear. Some trials indicate that estrogen improves function, as indicated by improvements in memory and attention. Current evidence from randomized controlled trials (RCTs) to support this effect is inadequate.

Urogenital

Women may experience a number of symptoms arising from the urogenital system around the menopause (Table 8.2).

Most of these symptoms are a result of atrophy of vaginal and urethral epithelium with loss of rugations and stenosis. A decreased maturation of cells leads to a decreased number of superficial cells.

There is a disturbance of the vaginal flora (decreased lactobacilli, increased fecal flora) and a resultant increase in vaginal pH. In the periurethral connective tissue there is a decreased amount of collagen.

Skeletal system

Bone mass reaches a peak in women toward the end of their third decade (see Fig. 8.2). It then remains relatively stable until menopause, at which time bone loss accelerates and is lifelong.

Table 8.2 Urogenital symptoms during menopause

Vaginal symptoms	Urinary symptoms
Vaginal dryness, irritation, discharge	Recurrent urinary tract infections
Vulvovaginal pruritus, pain	Urinary frequency, urgency
Dyspareunia	Dysuria, voiding difficulties
Postcoital bleeding	Urinary incontinence
Prolapse	
Anorgasmia	

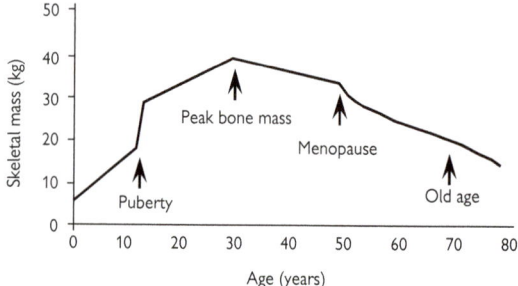

Figure 8.2 Bone density in women. Reproduced with permission from Birdwood GFB (1996). *Understanding Osteoporosis and Its Treatment: A Guide for Physicians and their Patients.* London: Taylor & Francis.

Some 70% of women over the age of 80 will have measurable osteoporosis (see Box 8.1). It is estimated that approximately 50% of Caucasian women will experience an osteoporosis-related fracture.

Cardiovascular risk

Coronary heart disease (CHD) is uncommon among premenopausal women, particularly if they do not smoke. There is a rapid increase in risk following menopause, with cardiovascular disease now being a leading cause of death among postmenopausal women.

The mechanism whereby premenopausal women have protection against CHD is not clear. However, it is known that estrogen has a number of protective effects:

- Nitric oxide–mediated vascular dilatation
- Inhibition of platelet aggregation
- Increased high-density lipoprotein (HDL), decreased low-density lipoprotein (LDL)
- Reduction in insulin resistance
- Antioxidant effect on endothelial cells
- Reduction in myocardial ischemia

The possible reduction in this increased risk of CHD in women on HRT after menopause was addressed in a large study, discussed in detail in the next section.

Box 8.1 Factors affecting bone mass and risk factors for fracture

Factors that can affect the bone mass

Affecting peak bone mass
- Genetic, racial
- Diet, calcium in adolescence

Affecting bone loss
- Premature menopause
- Amenorrhea
- Exercise, diet, weight
- Smoking, alcohol use, caffeine
- Use of corticosteroids

Risk factors that may affect the chance of fracture
- Low bone mass
  - Low body weight
  - Current cigarette smoking
- Personal or family history of fracture
- Risk factors for falls
  - Confusion disorders
  - Medications (sedative hypnotics, alcohol)
  - Neuromuscular disease
  - Environmental factors

Women's Health Initiative (WHI) trial

The WHI trial was set up with the primary aim of testing whether postmenopausal use of hormone replacement therapy (HRT) protected women from CHD.

The study was an RCT in which >16,000 American women were enrolled. The women were randomized to take placebo or HRT in the form of 0.625 mg of conjugated equine estrogens alone if the women had undergone hysterectomy or in conjunction with 2.5 mg of medroxyprogesterone acetate daily for those with a uterus.

The WHI chronicled women beyond the typical signs of the menopausal transition. The mean age was 64 years old. After 5 years of HRT treatment or nearly 7 years of estrogen replacement therapy (ERT), the following findings were reported:

1. A decrease in fracture
2. An increase in venus thromboembolic disease, primarily deep venous thrombosis (DVT) and not pulmonary embolism (PE)
3. An increase in cardiovascular disease, predominantly in those remote from the menopausal transition, with a protective effect in younger women using ERT.
4. No increase in breast cancer with estrogen use and a slight increase with HRT use (<1/1000)

Risks and benefits of HRT[1]

The Women's Health Initiative (WHI) was a study designed to determine the association between HRT and coronary heart disease post-menopause. The study found that taking estrogen-progestin in combination increases the risk of myocardial infraction (MI), breast cancer, thromboemboli, and stroke in postmenopausal women. Women who took estrogen alone only had an increased risk of stroke and thromboemboli with no increased risk of MI or breast cancer.

The study found that the risk of MI while on HRT is dependent on age, and that there was no increased risk in women who became menopausal less than 10 years before starting therapy or were between the ages of 50 and 59 while on therapy. Women who became menopausal more than 10 years before starting therapy or were over the age of 60 were at increased risk of having an MI, related to the therapy.

Women who took combined estrogen-progestin therapy had an increased risk of breast cancer, while women treated with estrogen alone had no risk.

There was an increased risk of developing dementia in women who took estrogen alone or combined estrogen-progestin, with no changes in memory or thinking. The risk of osteoporotic fractures was lower in women who took estrogen-progestin or estrogen alone. Both should not be used as preventative agents because bisphosphonates have fewer risks.

Multiple studies have shown that HRT can also decrease depression, but often antidepressants are needed for the patient to feel better.

---

[1] Barbieri RL, et al. (2010). Patient information: Postmenopausal hormone therapy. *UpToDate*.

HRT preparations

Estrogens are effective at relieving menopausal symptoms. For all women who have not had a hysterectomy, a progestogen should be added for at least 12 days of each month to prevent endometrial hyperplasia and carcinoma. The routes of administration of the estrogen can be

- Oral
- Patches
- Vaginal rings
- Gel
- Nasal spray

Oral regimens

These are well tolerated by many women, are cheaper, and are an appropriate first choice. Estrogen is given continuously, with progestogen either given continuously or added for at least 10 days per cycle in women with an intact uterus.

Fixed-dose combination preparations are convenient for patients not experiencing adverse effects and may improve compliance. Adjustment of the dose of individual hormones is possible by prescribing estrogen and progestogen separately.

Transdermal regimens

Women who experience nausea on oral therapy may tolerate a patch better. Transdermal regimens may also be considered for women with raised plasma triglycerides, gallbladder disease, or poor absorption. They are more expensive than oral regimens.

Topical preparations containing estrogen alone or containing estradiol in combination with progesterone are also available.

While reducing clotting factors, transfermals have not been shown to reduce DVT in a study using equivalent doses. Transdermals do not reduce cholesterol as well as oral preparations do.

Vaginal preparations

Vaginal estrogen creams and rings are indicated for atrophic vaginitis. They do not prevent osteoporosis. Long-term use by the vaginal route may be associated with endometrial hyperplasia, and additional oral progestogen should be given.

Regimens (Table 8.3)

The sequential regimens have estrogen in the first half of a 28-day cycle with progestogen in the second half. This is the appropriate regimen for women in the perimenopausal state. Continuous combined therapy of progestogen taken every day is useful for those women who are a few years past menopause and who do not wish to have any vaginal bleeding.

Side effects and complications of HRT

The main side effect is vaginal bleeding in women with a uterus. This can be decreased by the use of continuous combined therapy in women 2–3 years post-menopause.

Table 8.3 Suggested estrogen regimens

Perimenopausal women	Oral or transdermal cyclic estrogen plus cyclic progestogen
Nonsmoking perimenopausal women requiring contraception	Low-dose oral contraceptive until menopause, then HRT
Women 2–3 years postmenopause	Continuous estrogen-progestogen—oral or transdermal
Women who have had a hysterectomy	Continuous estrogen alone—oral or transdermal

The addition of progestogen in women with a uterus can cause bloating, fluid retention, and mastalgia. Progestogens can be administered vaginally as a cream or a suppository to try and reduce the severity of any side effects.

Venous thrombosis
There is a very small increased risk of venous thrombosis in women on HRT who do not have a previous history of venous thrombosis. The absolute risk has been approximated to 2/10,000 treatment years for venous thrombosis, 0.6/10,000 treatment years for pulmonary embolism, and 2/million treatment years for death.

The first 12 months of treatment are associated with the highest risk, however, at increased cost.

Alternative treatment

- Norethisterone 5 mg has been shown to be effective in reducing hot flashes and sweats, but it has little effect on other menopausal systems. Medroxyprogesterone acetate and megestrol work similarly.
- Propranolol and clonidine have been used for the treatment of hot flashes, but the effect is probably no better than placebo.
- Vaginal estrogen preparations can be used to treat atrophic vaginitis, but repeated use can lead to systematic absorption.
- Selective estrogen receptor modulators (SERMS) are effective in the prevention of bone loss and reduce the incidence of breast cancer. They may increase incidence of hot flashes slightly.
- Naturally occurring estrogens such as phytoestrogens occur in cereals and vegetables. Pharmaceutical preparations of these phytoestrogens have not been shown to be any better than placebo.

Chapter 9

Initial advice regarding delays in conception

Prevalence of fertility problems *84*
Timing of the initial investigation *84*
Female partner's age *85*
Frequency and timing of intercourse *85*
Environmental and dietary influences *86*

Prevalence of fertility problems

Sixteen percent of couples fail to conceive after 1 year of unprotected regular intercourse. After 2 years, with no treatment, about half of these couples will still not have conceived and, after a further year, ~7% in all will remain infertile.

Most couples will turn for help after 1 year. That means that one in seven couples will look for advice after 1 year. Women over the age of 35 should consider seeking evaluation after 6 months of failure to conceive.

Timing of the initial investigation

Couples who have not succeeded in conceiving after 1 year of regular unprotected intercourse should be offered investigation of the failure to conceive.

Earlier investigation and treatment should be initiated when there is a history of obvious fertility-impeding factors, such as oligo- or amenorrhea, previous pelvic surgical intervention, previous ectopic pregnancy, pelvic inflammatory disease (PID), undescended testis, sexual dysfunction, a history of cancer treatment, or if the female partner is ≥35 years of age.

At all consultations, both partners should be present if possible.

Female partner's age

Advancing female age is probably the single most important factor influencing fertility potential. Physiologically, from the age of ~35 years and older, there is a steady downward trend in fertility capacity. This is probably a reflection of the declining number of primordial follicles remaining, biological aging, and exposure to many deleterious influences on the ova remaining in the ovaries.

In addition to the persistently decreasing number of available, potentially fertilizable oocytes, it is also assumed that the best quality ova are preferentially recruited in the earlier stages of the reproductive period. As a result, from the mid-30s, fertility potential decreases considerably, and after the age of 42, a spontaneous pregnancy becomes quite a rare event.

Advancing female age affects not only natural conception but also the results of ovulation induction and assisted reproductive technologies.

Public awareness of these facts is insufficient. Many women, with a delayed wish for conception or aspiring to be single mothers, and with increasing divorce rates and second marriages, do not comprehend the profound effect of advancing female age on fertility potential. The medical profession has not yet succeeded in impressing on the general public the importance of these facts. An awareness of declining pregnancy rates with age at least allows an informed consideration of the timing of attempted conception when this is flexible.

In order to inform couples fully of their prognosis regarding fertility potential, especially if the female partner is in the more advanced age group, data on the state of ovarian function are needed. This information should be used to not only forecast the chances of conception but also to decide whether treatment should be embarked upon at all.

To answer these questions, information on the number of available oocytes (ovarian reserve) and their quality is needed. Tests of ovarian reserve include day 3 FSH and estradiol, inhibin B, anti-Müllerian hormone, and antral follicle count, as well as dynamic tests such as clomifene challenge test. The results of the tests available require accurate interpretation of their value before any informed discussion can be undertaken.

Frequency and timing of intercourse

Many couples attempting to conceive are unaware that regular intercourse around the time of ovulation is a basic requirement. Trite as this may sound, a simple explanation of the approximate time of presumed ovulation for the woman with regular cycles may prove very helpful.

If the couple is advised to have intercourse a minimum of once every 2 days around this time, pregnancies can be achieved in many cases without further investigation or treatment.

Intercourse may be timed according to ovulation by the use of urinary ovulation predictor kits, which are widely available. Intercourse should occur when the kit demonstrates ovulation is imminent.

Environmental and dietary influences

Alcohol
Excessive regular alcohol consumption by the male partner may affect not only sexual performance but also semen quality.

Smoking
The habit of smoking is clearly not good for general health, and couples attempting to conceive should be encouraged to stop smoking. There is evidence to show that women who smoke heavily may have a reduced fertility potential and that the semen quality of men who smoke may be reduced.

Occupation
The occupations of the couple concerned about their fertility should be noted. Occupations such as long-distance truck or bus driving in hot climates, those involving exposure to bromide or similar chemicals, or work involving exposure to irradiation have all been associated with a decrease in fertility potential.

Medications
Many medications, whether prescribed or over the counter, and recreational drugs may interfere with male and female infertility. Patients need to be informed of the potential effects of such medications and appropriate measures should be taken. Some of the most common examples include sedatives that increase prolactin discharge, so-called complementary medications containing estrogens, and salazopyrines that may have drastic effects on semen quality.

Body weight
Both extremes of body weight may have a significant effect on fertility potential. Obese women (body mass index [BMI] ≥30), especially those with associated anovulation, have a significant disadvantage in fertility potential. They take longer to conceive, require more drugs for ovarian stimulation, and are at a greater risk of miscarriage than those of normal weight. Participation in a program involving instruction in diet, weight loss and exercise is advised.

Obese men are also more likely to have reduced fertility and should also be encouraged to lose weight. Underweight women (BMI <19) who have oligo- or amenorrhea should be encouraged to increase their weight, as often this alone may restore regular ovulation.

Folic acid supplementation
Every woman intending to conceive should be advised to take folic acid, 400 micrograms/day, before conception and up to 12 weeks into the pregnancy. This has been shown significantly to reduce the risk of having a baby with a neural tube defect.

For women who have previously had an infant with a neural tube defect or who are receiving antiepileptic medication, a higher dose of 5 mg/day is recommended.

Chapter 10

Defining infertility

Introduction 88
General points before starting investigation 89

Introduction

Infertility, for practical purposes, may be regarded as a failure to conceive following at least 1 year of regular unprotected sexual intercourse. In the general population, the prevalence is 16% after 1 year but 8% after 2 years (Fig. 10.1).

This is known as *primary infertility* if the woman has had no previous pregnancies. When the couple has had a previous child or children and has failed to conceive following at least 1 year of regular unprotected sexual intercourse, this is defined as *secondary infertility*.

- The prevalence of infertility varies with age and is 5.5, 9.4 and 19.7%, respectively, at ages 25–29, 30–34, and 35–39 years.
- Most couples will turn to help after 1 year, i.e., 1 in 7 couples will look for advice after 1 year.

Intervention involving initial investigation of the cause of the infertility is unjustified before at least 1 year has passed. There are several exceptions to this rule. Early intervention is indicated when a simple history reveals one of the following obviously fertility-related symptoms:

- Female age >35 years
- Menstrual irregularity, not within the limits of a 24- to 35-day cycle
- Previous pelvic or testicular surgical intervention for ectopic pregnancy, ovarian cystectomy, ruptured appendix, or undescended testis
- History of pelvic inflammatory disease (PID) or sexually transmitted diseases (STDs)
- Known endometriosis
- Fertility treatment was required to attain a previous pregnancy
- Sexual problems precluding regular normal intercourse
- Previous ectopic pregnancy
- History of cancer treatment in male or female
- Male genital trauma

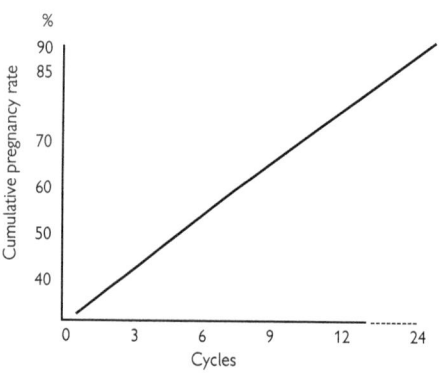

Figure 10.1 Cumulative conception rates according to the number of cycles of attempted conception in the general population.

General points before starting investigation

- Infertility is the problem of a couple, and wherever possible, both members should be involved in clinic visits and decision making. Apportioning blame to one or the other person should be avoided.
- Infertility is a stressful situation. Sympathetic handling, full explanations, and encouragement are essential components of the management.
- A basic explanation of the timing of intercourse in relation to the probable time of ovulation can be very helpful to the couple.
- Overweight and obesity are obstacles to attaining a pregnancy and are also associated with an increased incidence of spontaneous miscarriage. Advice on the importance of these facts and the necessary information for their correction should be given before any treatment is initiated. Warnings about impairment of fertility function through excessive alcohol intake, cigarette smoking, and drug abuse should also be given at this stage, when relevant.
- Every woman attempting conception should be given folic acid, 0.4 mg daily, to prevent neural tube defects in the infant. This should be continued until at least the 12th week of the pregnancy.
- Fertility potential, in general, starts to decline after the age of 35 years in the female. Delay in the decision to conceive beyond this age and especially over the age of 39, an increasing trend in the modern world, can create serious problems. Couples should be well informed of this situation when discussing the decision to have a child.

Chapter 11

Investigation of fertility problems

Introduction *92*
Investigation of the male partner *95*
Investigation of the female partner *98*
Investigation of a possible mechanical factor *100*
Further reading *102*

Introduction

The aim of the investigation of the infertile couple is to find the cause(s) of the problem and treat accordingly. Both investigation and treatment are logical stepwise processes (see Fig. 11.1 and Fig. 11.2, pp. 92 and 93). A disorganized approach may sometimes be successful, but it is not the most efficient, safe, and economical way to approach the problem.

Accurate history-taking is absolutely essential for discerning the cause(s) of the infertility. By listening carefully and asking direct questions, many

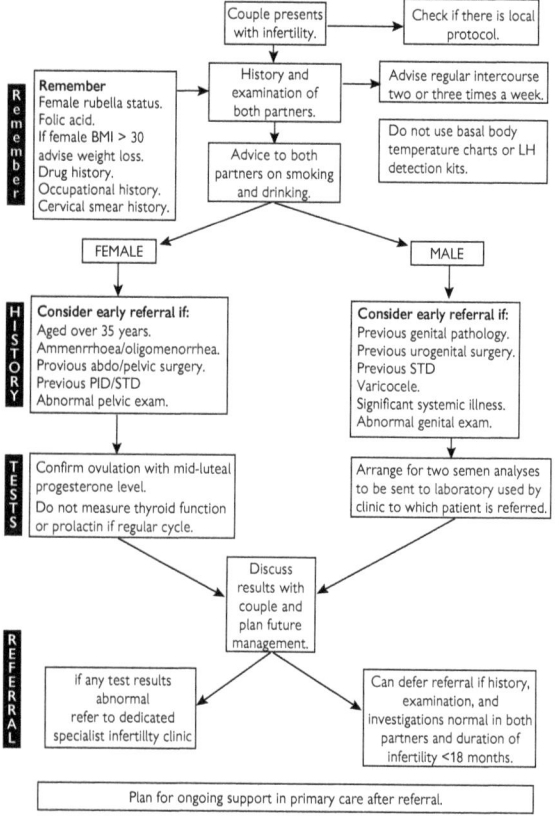

Figure 11.1 Initial investigation of the couple at the primary care level.

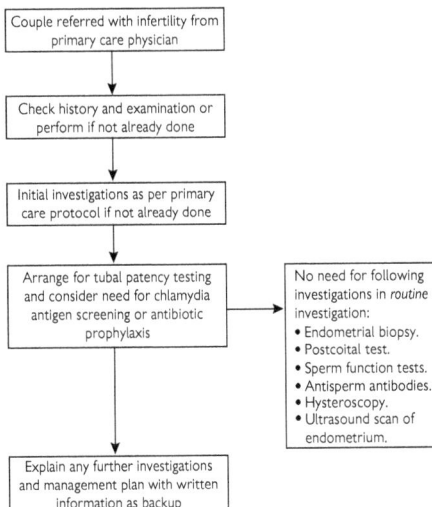

Figure 11.2 Initial investigation and management of the couple in secondary care.

clues can be found. A suggested checklist for the female partner is presented in Table 7.2. The headings can be used as a guide at the first consultation. The answers to the direct questions can prompt further, more detailed inquiries, e.g. is the amenorrhea primary or secondary? If primary, is there a problem with the sense of smell? If secondary, are there any hot flashes?

A thorough gynecological and general examination should also be performed at the first visit. Again, a suggested checklist is provided in Table 7.2. For history-taking and examination of the male partner, see the next section.

The results of the history and examination alone will often indicate the possible cause of the infertility and will dictate the order in which the more specific examinations should be made. Many couples may have more than one specific cause for their infertility, and up to 30% of cases may be "unexplained" in that all of the basic and more specific infertility investigations prove to be normal.

The investigation of the infertile couple at a basic, first-line level involves a semen analysis and an examination of ovulatory function and the integrity of the female reproductive tract. An abnormal result for any of these basic investigations may prompt second-line examinations.

Table 11.1 sets out possible first- and second-line examinations that are commonly used.

CHAPTER 11 Investigation of fertility problems

Table 11.1 Possible first- and second-line examinations for the investigation of fertility

	Ovulation, ovarian reserve	Mechanical	Male
First-line	History, day 3 FSH, urinary LH	HSG	Semen analysis
Second-line	LH, T, PROL, TSH Androgens in serum	Laparoscopy Hysteroscopy Tubal catheter	Physical exam; FSH; test LH, TSH, PRL

FSH, follicle-stimulating hormone; HSG, hysterosalpingography; LH, luteinizing hormone; PROL, prolactin; T, testosterone; TSH, thyroid-stimulating hormone.

Investigation of the male partner

A semen analysis should be performed in every case of infertility as a routine screening test. The semen is produced by masturbation and the fresh sperm should be examined within 30 minutes. It has become traditional to request abstinence from ejaculation for 2–3 days before obtaining the sample. Abstinence of >5 days before sampling may result in decreased sperm motility.

Normal parameters of a semen sample are listed in Table 11.2. The standard criteria are those of the WHO (2000), but for the analysis of sperm morphology, Kruger's strict criteria have been added and are now widely used. Sperm motility is graded according to progressive forward motility, grade a (≥25% rapid progressive motility) or grade b (slow or sluggish progressive motility) or, alternatively, from grade I, fast forward; grade II, slow forward; grade III, minimal forward progression; to grade IV, no motility.

A reduced sperm concentration, *oligospermia*, is often accompanied by reduced sperm motility, *asthenospermia*. More detailed information regarding sperm motility can be obtained by using a computerized image analysis system, which is said to correlate well with the fertilizing capacity of the sperm.

Kruger's strict criteria are recommended for the assessment of sperm morphology. According to these criteria, <14% normal forms, *teratozoospermia*, carries a poor prognosis for fertilization.

A completely normal semen analysis indicates that no further examination is needed and, practically, that no further investigation of the male partner is required. An abnormal semen analysis necessitates a repeat examination,

Table 11.2 WHO reference values for semen analysis (2000): normal parameters of a semen sample

Volume: 2.0 mL or more
Liquefaction time: Within 60 minutes
pH: 7.2 or more
Concentration: 20 million spermatozoa/mL or more
Total sperm number: 40 million spermatozoa per ejaculate or more
Motility: 50% or more (grades a* and b**) or 25% with progressive forward motility (grade a*)
Vitality: 75% or more live
White blood cells: fewer than 1 million/mL
Morphology: >30% normal forms (WHO) >14% normal forms (Kruger strict criteria)

* Grade a = rapid progressive motility (sperm moving swiftly, usually in a straight line).

** Grade b = slow or sluggish progressive motility (sperm may be less linear in their progression).

best done 3 months later, before any therapeutic decisions are made; a single-sample analysis will falsely identify ~10% of men as abnormal, but repeating the test reduces this to 2%.

Theoretically, a full history and examination of the male partner should be taken at the first clinic visit. In practice, obviously relevant history (e.g., undescended testis, orchitis) is noted at this time, but the rest of the detailed history and physical examination is usually only performed following an abnormal semen analysis.

History
- Medical—onset of puberty, diabetes mellitus, cystic fibrosis, past history of mumps, orchitis, STDs, anosmia
- Surgical—maldescended testis, hernia repair, varicocele
- Family history—genetic diseases
- Medications—including anabolic steroids
- Occupation—exposure to excessive heat or chemicals, excessive physical activity
- Abuse—drugs, alcohol, smoking

Examination
- *Androgenicity*—hair distribution, voice, body build, gynecomastia
- *Testicular size*—if abnormal can be quantified with an orchidometer (Prader beads). The normal range is 12–30 mL. Testicular consistency
- Undescended testis, spermatocele, varicocele, absence of the vas deferens
- *Rectal examination*—palpation of the prostate gland, prostatic massage to obtain a urethral secretion for culture

Further examinations

Hormonal
Serum concentrations of LH, FSH, testosterone, estradiol, and prolactin should be measured. Hormone concentrations are principally of use for confirming suspected diagnoses of hypogonadotropic hypogonadism (very low gonadotropins) or of testicular failure when gonadotropins are high and testosterone is low.

Chromosome analysis
Klinefelter's syndrome (47, XXY) should be suspected if the testes are small and firm.

Imaging of the testes
This includes ultrasound, isotopic examination of testicular blood flow for a suspected varicocele, and a vasogram if there is suspicion of obstructive azospermia (normal-sized testes with normal hormonal concentrations).

Postcoital test (PCT)
A PCT, performed during the immediate preovulatory period ~10 hours after intercourse, entails examining retrieved cervical mucous under a microscope for the presence and movement of sperm. It is only really useful when positive—i.e., the presence of ≥10 motile sperm per microscopic

low-power field is reassuring that intercourse is successfully depositing motile sperm in receptive cervical mucous.

A complete absence of sperm could indicate a faulty coital technique, azospermia, or hostile cervical mucous. The absence of sperm motility could indicate a hostile cervical mucous or asthenospermia.

Most reproductive endocrinologists no longer employ the PCT as a routine examination because of its limited yield of useful information.

The management of male infertility can be found in Chapter 13; information on intrauterine insemination is presented in Chapter 17. Intracytoplasmic sperm injection and donor insemination are discussed in Chapter 18.

A urinary LH kit may be used to ensure an LH surge and is also useful to time ovulation and intercourse. The kit is inexpensive, widely available, without prescription, and easy to use. An early-morning urine sample should be used.

Screening should start cycle day 10 in a woman with a regular 28-day cycle and continue until ovulation. A positive response at mid-cycle indicates a high probability of normal ovulation.

Investigation of the female partner

The investigation of the female partner basically consists of an examination of ovulatory function and the mechanical integrity of the reproductive tract. While ovulatory function is relatively easy to assess, investigation of a mechanical factor is more invasive. Nonetheless, it is a common condition and should not be delayed.

Ovulatory function

Any form of menstrual irregularity, not within the limits of a 24- to 35-day cycle, strongly suggests a diagnosis of anovulation or oligo-ovulation. The converse is not always true, as the occasional woman with regular cycles may be anovulatory. Premenstrual molimina (breast tenderness, bloating, and mood changes) usually indicates that ovulation is occurring.

For confirmation that ovulation is occurring, four possible methods are used: plasma progesterone concentrations, a basal body temperature (BBT) chart, vaginal ultrasound examination, and urinary LH kits.

Plasma progesterone concentrations are arguably the most accurate way to estimate whether ovulation has occurred. For women with a regular cycle of 28 days, a plasma progesterone estimation on cycle day 20 or 21 of ≥8 ng/mL (25nmol/L) will rule out a diagnosis of anovulation. If the usual cycle is 35 days in length, then this examination should be done around cycle day 28, i.e., ~7 days before the expected menstruation.

For women with mild oligomenorrhea (cycle length >35 days), progesterone can be measured on day 28 and then once a week until menstruation occurs. If periods only occur less than once every 2 months or in cases of secondary amenorrhea, there is little point in hunting for progesterone estimations as the diagnosis of severe oligo- or anovulation is self-apparent.

The principle of the BBT chart in estimating whether ovulation is occurring is that the secretion of progesterone, following ovulation, into the circulation will cause a rise in body temperature of ~0.5°C. The typical BBT chart will thus be biphasic, i.e., the temperature following ovulation will be higher than that in the first part or follicular phase. The day before the temperature rise is usually denoted as the day of ovulation.

Although the BBT is a simple, cheap, and noninvasive screening test, it suffers from many inaccuracies, particularly false negatives, and is open to much misinterpretation. It is very doubtful whether the BBT still has a place in the routine screening for ovulatory problems. Further, it has been found to be a nuisance for many women, as body temperature must be measured every morning, immediately on waking.

A vaginal ultrasound examination before and after ovulation should record a large, developing, dominant follicle that disappears following ovulation. In addition, most competent ultrasonographers are able to diagnose the presence of a corpus luteum if ovulation has occurred. This may be accompanied by a small amount of fluid in the pouch of Douglas.

Physical examination can give many clues as to the cause of anovulation. Most obvious at first glance is the weight of the patient. Weight and height should always be recorded and the body mass index (BMI) calculated. This is done with the following formula:

$$BMI = \frac{\text{Weight (kg)}}{\text{Height in meters}^2}$$

- A normal BMI is 20–25.
- <20 is underweight.
- 25.1–30 is overweight.
- >30 is frank obesity.

Some geographical variations in these diagnoses exist. For example, in most Southeast Asian communities, any BMI >25 is regarded as obesity.

Overweight and obesity
Overweight and obesity are often associated with polycycstic ovary syndrome (PCOS), and PCOS is often characterized by hirsutism and/or acne, both of which are easily discernible on examination.

In women with suspected PCOS who are obese, acanthosis nigricans, dark discoloration of the skin in the axillary or nuchal regions, is a telltale sign of insulin resistance. Waist circumference should be measured at the level between the umbilicus and the iliac crests in all overweight women, as this again may be a good reflection of insulin resistance when >88 cm.

Weight-related amenorrhea
Women whose BMI is <20 may have irregular or absent ovulation related to weight-related amenorrhea. This may be due to loss of weight from dieting and anorexia nervosa or exercise in its extreme.

Direct questioning about diet, alcohol use, or drug abuse is mandatory.

Estrogen deficiency
Physical examination can also reveal signs of estrogen deficiency, such as poor breast development, lack of development of the vulva, vaginal dryness, and lack of additional secondary sexual characteristics. These signs indicating estrogen deprivation could be due to either hypo- or hypergonadotropic hypogonadism when either is associated with primary amenorrhea.

Although Turner's syndrome is a rare cause of amenorrhea, it can often be easily diagnosed by the typical body habitus: short stature, webbed neck, cubitus valgus, and often a systolic cardiac murmur.

Distribution of hair growth
Distribution of hair growth should be noted. A male distribution would indicate hyperandrogenism, and a lack of body hair could be a sign of androgen insensitivity. Clitoral enlargement or lack of development would occur parallel to these respective conditions in their extreme.

Once the diagnosis of oligo- or anovulation has been established, further investigation is required to find the cause. Full details of the classification of ovulatory disorders and their investigation are described in Chapter 7.

Investigation of a possible mechanical factor

X-ray hysterosalpingography (HSG)

If there is a previous history of STD in the female partner, a complicated delivery, Caesarean section, previous ectopic pregnancy, PID, endometriosis, or surgical interventions in the pelvic region, including appendectomy, a screening test, usually X-ray HSG, should be performed. An HSG should also be performed if both semen analysis and ovulatory function are normal.

The HSG is a diagnostic procedure in which the cervical canal, uterine cavity, and lumina of the fallopian tubes are radiographically visualized by the injection of radio-opaque contrast medium through a cervical cannula. HSG is capable of demonstrating congenital uterine abnormalities, intrauterine lesions such as polyps, fibroids, and adhesions, and patency and abnormalities of the fallopian tubes.

Iodine sensitivity is a contraindication. An HSG should not be performed during uterine bleeding, to avoid intravasation, and not in the luteal phase of the cycle, to avoid the possible presence of an early pregnancy.

Water-soluble media are now used in preference to oil-based media, as the latter carry a risk of intravasation and possible embolism. The injection of up to 5 mL of contrast medium, usually water-soluble, is often enough to obtain all the information needed. The use of larger than necessary volumes may produce discomfort and may obscure lesions in the uterine cavity.

The demonstration of a normal uterine cavity on HSG obviates the need for hysteroscopy, which may be used for the confirmation and possible operative removal of lesions within the uterine cavity demonstrated on HSG. Some centers use laparoscopy as a screening test if the history is suggestive of a possible mechanical factor, but HSG serves this purpose well and is certainly a less invasive technique. If HSG is suggestive of a tubal lesion or peritubal adhesions, or when significant pelvic adhesions are suspected, then laparoscopy is performed.

If the HSG confirms tubal patency and a normal uterine cavity, then usually no further workup to diagnose a mechanical factor cause of the infertility is needed at the screening stage. Abnormal findings in the HSG will dictate what further steps should be taken. These may include a diagnostic laparoscopy and hysteroscopy, which may be diagnostic or operative, or gross tubal damage demonstrated on the HSG, such as sactosalpinx, may indicate direct progress to in vitro fertilization (IVF).

Although HSG should be used as a purely diagnostic procedure, there is some evidence of a possible therapeutic effect in patients with apparently normal patent fallopian tubes. Following an HSG with water-soluble contrast medium, more pregnancies result than would be expected to occur spontaneously when not performing an HSG. This may be due to the separation of "sticky" fimbria, mild peritubal adhesions or tubal plugs.

Ultrasound

Sonohysterography or saline-infused sonohystogram (SIS) is the infusion of saline into the uterus during sonography. It is simple, cheap, minimally invasive, and relatively painless and avoids the use of hysteroscopy or radiation for obtaining information principally about the uterine cavity.

However, given the limitations of sonohysterography, mainly its inability to visualize tubal patency directly, HSG remains the gold standard for routine screening for infertility and hysteroscopy for direct visualization of the uterine cavity.

Sonosalpingography, employing a contrast medium, has not proven to be as accurate as HSG.

Laparoscopy

Laparoscopy entails the controlled introduction of carbon dioxide into the peritoneal cavity in order to distend it and enable visualization by the introduction of the laparoscope. For the investigation of infertility, a blue dye is injected through the cervical canal to assess tubal patency and free flow into the pelvic cavity.

A full assessment of the pelvis should be made on laparoscopy, including the peritoneal surface of the uterus, bladder, appendix, and bowel. Endometriosis can be spotted and mapped, and an inspection of the ovaries can reveal the presence of cysts, polycystic ovaries, normally developing follicles, and signs of ovulation.

Following a thorough inspection of the pelvis, blue dye is injected through a cervical cannula. Evidence of its passage from both distal ends of the tubes should be sought as well as its free flow into the pelvic cavity. The presence of pelvic adhesions can be noted and, if thin and flimsy, they can easily be separated during the diagnostic procedure.

The advantages of laparoscopy and dye injection over HSG as a diagnostic procedure are that laparoscopy allows full visualization of the pelvic cavity and can diagnose the presence of endometriosis, pelvic adhesions, particularly peritubal and para-ovarian adhesions, and other pelvic pathology. Furthermore, some of these conditions can be treated during the same procedure.

Laparoscopy is also usually capable of overcoming tubal spasm, which is sometimes a cause of a false diagnosis of proximal tubal occlusion on HSG. However, laparoscopy cannot give information on the uterine cavity; for this reason, many units combine a diagnostic laparoscopy with hysteroscopy at the same sitting.

The disadvantages of laparoscopy are that it is an invasive procedure that may cause morbidity such as anesthetic complications, perforation of an abdominal viscus, or hemorrhage. It also carries a 1:12,000 risk of mortality.

Although some centers employ laparoscopy as a first-line procedure for the investigation of infertility in patients thought to have co-morbidities, it is more commonly used for confirmation of abnormalities seen on HSG for clarifying unexplained infertility or for the diagnosis and extent of suspected endometriosis.

Further reading

ACOG Infertility Bulletin. (2002). Management of infertility caused by ovulatory dysfunction. *Obstet Gynecol*. 99(2):347–358.

Collins JA (1988). Diagnostic assessment of the infertile female partner. *Curr Probl Obstet Gynecol Fertil* 11:6–42.

Rowe PJ, Comhaire FH, Hargreave TB, Mahmoud AM (2000). *WHO Manual for the Standardized Investigation, Diagnosis and Management of the Infertile Male*. Cambridge, UK: Cambridge University Press, 2000.

Chapter 12

Management strategies for fertility problems

Principles *104*
Management of investigations *105*
Management strategies *106*

Principles

- People who have not conceived following 1 year of regular unprotected intercourse should be offered investigations of the inability to conceive.
- Earlier investigation may be offered when predisposing factors causing infertility become obvious from history-taking, e.g., oligo- or amenorrhea, pelvic inflammatory disease (PID), pelvic surgery, endometriosis, ectopic pregnancy, or undescended testis, or when female age is ≥35 years.
- Whenever possible, couples experiencing problems conceiving should be seen together. This is to emphasize the fact that the problem is of a couple rather than of an individual.
- Full explanations of investigations and treatment, with available additional counseling, can do much to alleviate the stress associated with fertility problems.
- The secondary management of infertility problems is a specialist subject and should ideally be performed by a reproductive endocrinologist or gynecologist with expertise in infertility evaluation and treatment.

Management of investigations

The basic investigation of fertility problems should always include a semen analysis and assessment of ovulation.

A normal semen analysis (see Table 11.2) precludes the need for further examination. A grossly abnormal result (azoospermia or severe oligo-terato-asthenospermia) necessitates a repeat test without further delay. An otherwise abnormal result should be confirmed or negated by a repeat test after 3 months, as this is the normal duration of a sperm cycle.

The practical help from the performance of a screening test for anti-sperm antibodies is doubtful. The further investigation of an abnormal semen analysis is described in detail in Chapter 11.

Ovulation can be most simply confirmed in women with regular cycles by measuring serum progesterone concentration in the mid-luteal phase, i.e., day 21 in a woman with 28-day cycles. A serum progesterone concentration of >5 ng/mL (25 nmol/L) is a clear indication that ovulation is occurring.

For women with prolonged cycles, a similar blood test should be performed ~7 days before the time of the expected menstruation. For women age ≥35 years, a routine examination of serum FSH, estradiol, and LH is warranted on day 3 of the cycle. For the further investigation of oligo- or anovulation, see Chapter 7.

A history of conditions such as PID, pelvic surgery (including appendectomy), previous Caesarean section, ectopic pregnancy, or endometriosis indicates early investigation of a possible mechanical factor. In the absence of any hint of a mechanical problem, its assessment can be left to a later stage if needed, preferably by hysterosalpingography (HSG).

Some clinicians prefer performing a laparoscopy using a dye as the first-line investigation, but this is a more invasive examination and should be reserved for when an HSG reveals obvious abnormalities. Further, the use of an HSG as a screening test, as opposed to laparoscopy, has the advantage of showing the uterine cavity. The revelation of clear evidence of a lesion, e.g., bilateral tubal occlusion with hydrosalpinges, can indicate proceeding directly to IVF or tubal surgery, without the need to perform a diagnostic laparoscopy.

For a more detailed discussion of investigation of a mechanical factor, see Chapter 11.

Management strategies

The basic history, examination, and investigations will point to one or more diagnostic categories that will indicate the line of treatment to be employed. These are described only briefly here but more fully in the relevant individual chapters.

Alternatively, no firm diagnosis may have been made following first- and second-line investigations (unexplained or idiopathic infertility). This "diagnosis," or lack of diagnosis, will be dealt with more fully below.

Although divided here into male infertility, ovulatory, and mechanical defects, it is not uncommon to unveil any combination of these, so-called multifactorial infertility. Similarly, the same line of treatment may be applied for different conditions.

Tables 12.1–12.4 list treatment possibilities according to the presumed diagnostic category and point out the relevant chapters containing detailed descriptions of the various treatment modes.

Male infertility

Table 12.1 lists possible treatment modes according to the various causes of sperm defects. This list is only a rough guide as, for example, the source of oligo-terato-asthenospermia is largely idiopathic. Moreover, many of

Table 12.1 Treatment possibilities for male fertility problems

- General health—limit alcohol, tobacco smoking, recreational drugs
  - Avoid sulfasalazine, cimetidine, calcium antagonists
  - Occupational toxins
- Hypogonadotropic-hypogonadism—gonadotropins, pulsatile GnRH (see Chapter 13)
- Mild oligo-terato-asthenospermia—intrauterine insemination (see Chapter 17)
- Severe oligo-terato-asthenospermia—IVF/ICSI (see Chapter 18)
- Obstructive azospermia—TESE, MESA, or PESA + IVF/ICSI
  - Surgical correction, where relevant (see Chapter 13)
- Hypergonadotropic testicular failure—TESE, MESA, or PESA + IVF/ICSI
- Absolute azospermia or genetic disease—donor insemination. (see Chapter 13)
- Leukospermia, prostatitis—antibiotics (see Chapter 13)
- Retrograde ejaculation—washing of sperm after recovery from urine
- Varicocele, grade III and IV—ligation of spermatic vein (controversial)
- Erectile failure—sildenafil, tadalafil.
- Vasectomy—reversal or PESA

GnRH, gonadotropin-releasing hormone; ICSI, intracytoplasmic injection; IVF, in vitro fertilization; MESA, microsurgical epididymal sperm aspiration; PESA, percutaneous epididymal sperm aspiration; TESE, testicular sperm extraction.

the treatment modes are suitable for different conditions, and often the appropriate treatment is determined by the severity of sperm defect rather than by the underlying cause, whether known or not.

The vast majority of sperm defects causing infertility are treated by either intrauterine insemination (IUI) for the milder cases of oligo-teratoasthenospermia or intracytoplasmatic sperm injection (ICSI) for the rest.

General health recommendations can, at best, only marginally improve sperm function, and the value of treatment with antibiotics for leucospermia and ligation of the spermatic vein(s) to repair varicocele is still being disputed.

The diagnoses of hypogonadotropic hypogonadism and obstructive azoospermia are relatively rare and together account for <3% of all cases of male infertility. In contrast, nonobstructive azoospermia and severe oligospermia due to testicular failure are common, and the cause is often unknown.

For details of the treatment modes listed in Table 12.1, the reader is referred to the relevant chapters indicated in the table.

Ovulatory dysfunction

The treatment of ovulatory dysfunction (see Table 12.2) caused by hypothalamic–pituitary failure (WHO Group I), ovarian failure (Group III), and hyperprolactinemia (Group IV) are clearly defined; details can be found in Chapter 14.

The treatment of hypothalamic–pituitary dysfunction (almost entirely due to PCOS), in contrast, offers a plethora of alternatives. Details of when and how to employ these treatments are given in Chapters 5 (PCOS) and 14 (Ovulation induction) and include algorithms.

Table 12.2 Treatment possibilities for anovulation or oligo-ovulation

- Hypothalamic–pituitary failure (WHO Group I)—gonadotropins, pulsatile GnRH (see Chapters 7 and 14)
- Hypothalamic–pituitary dysfunction (Group II) (see Chapters 5 and 14)
  - Lifestyle changes
  - Clomifene citrate
  - Aromatase inhibitors
  - Metformin
  - Low-dose FSH or hMG
  - Laparoscopic ovarian drilling
  - IVF
  - In vitro maturation of oocytes
- Ovarian failure (Group III)—ovum donation (see Chapter 18)
- Hyperprolactinemia (Group IV)—dopamine agonists (see Chapter 14)

Mechanical factors in the female partner

Most of these disorders (see Table 12.3) should be treated by IVF or embryo transfer (ET). A few specialized centers in tubal surgery obtain excellent results from anastomosis following tubal ligation. Much depends on the type and extent of the lesion.

However, tubal occlusion caused by infection tends to negatively affect tubal function and not merely patency; in these cases, IVF is the preferred treatment. Moreover, the presence of hydrosalpinx, whether unilateral or bilateral, suspected on HSG and confirmed by ultrasound examination or seen on laparoscopy, negatively affects the outcome of IVF.

Salpingectomy preceding IVF improves results considerably. Tubal patency can be restored in cases of proximal tubal occlusion by tubal catheterization. Details of all these modes of treatment can be found in Chapters 15 and 18. The management of endometriosis causing infertility is described in Chapter 16.

Unexplained fertility

Unexplained (idiopathic) infertility is a diagnosis of exclusion. It is estimated that the label of unexplained infertility is attached to a couple in up to 30% of all cases presenting with infertility, depending on the duration of the infertility.

Couples are often labeled as "unexplained infertility" following 1 year of regular, unprotected intercourse when tests for ovulation and tubal patency and a semen analysis are all normal.

The high prevalence of unexplained infertility is a reminder of the lack of accuracy and subtlety of the diagnostic examinations employed. For example, tubal patency does not necessarily indicate normal tubal function; a normal routine semen examination tells us little about the functional capacity of the sperm and the subtleties of zona penetration; and proof of ovulation tells us nothing about the quality of the ovum.

The decision of when to intervene for the treatment of unexplained infertility is influenced by the age of the female partner, the duration of infertility, and the attitude adopted by both the physician and patients. After 1 year of unexplained infertility in a woman of ≥35 years, treatment intervention should not be delayed.

Table 12.3 Treatment possibilities for female mechanical factor infertility (see Chapters 15 and 18)

- Tubal occlusion—IVF/ET
- Hydrosalpinx—IVF/ET, preceded by salpingectomy
- Distal tubal occlusion— IVF/ET, possible fimbrioplasty
- Peritubal/periovarian adhesions—laparoscopic adhesiolysis
- Proximal tubal occlusion— IVF/ET, tubal catheterization, operative hysteroscopy
- Moderate to severe endometriosis—surgical ablation (see Chapter 16)

Table 12.4 Treatment possibilities for unexplained infertility (see also Chapters 17 and 18)

- Expectant treatment
- Clomifene citrate ± IUI
- IUI—unstimulated cycle
- IUI with gonadotropin stimulation
- IVF/ET

Table 12.4 lists possible treatment modes for unexplained infertility, all of which are necessarily empirical. They are listed in the usual order, from the "easy" to the more difficult.

In practice, IUI alone or clomifene citrate alone fare only marginally better than expectant treatment. The combination of gonadotropin stimulation and IUI is considerably more successful in terms of pregnancy rates. However, caution is advised regarding the high incidence of multiple pregnancies with this method. A full discussion can be found in Chapter 17.

IVF is usually performed last in these patients, usually after 3–6 cycles of stimulated cycles and IUI. IVF may uncover an explanation for the infertility by revealing a lack of fertilization due to either an egg or sperm defect, previously unsuspected. Therefore, a more rapid program to IVF may be indicated, especially in those over 35 years of age.

Chapter 13

Male infertility

Introduction *112*
Etiology *113*
Investigation of the male *116*
Further reading *120*

Introduction

Other than in cases of absolute azoospermia or severe oligospermia or asthenospermia, the impact of a male factor on a couple's infertility is difficult to quantify. Indeed, as can be seen in men after a vasectomy, when extremely small amounts of motile sperm can be present, conception can occur. Accepting this "male factor" may be a contributing if not absolute factor in >25% of cases of subfertility.

Etiology

Primary testicular disease

Most cases of male infertility lie in this category. In >50% of cases, no obvious predisposing factor can be identified. Y chromosome microdeletions are common in 10–15% of men with azoospermia or severe oligospermia.

These microdeletions are too small to be detected by karyotyping. They can be easily identified using polymerase chain reaction (PCR).

Most of the microdeletions that cause azoospermia or oligospermia occur in the nonoverlapping regions of the long arm of the Y chromsome. These regions, also called azoospermia factor regions, are responsible for spermatogenesis. The loci are termed AZFa, AZFb and AZFc from proximal to distal Yq (Yq11.21–23 region).

Several genes located in AZF regions are associated with spermatogenesis (see Fig. 13.1).

> **Other causes of failure of spermatogenesis**
> - Testicular maldescent
> - Testicular torsion
> - Trauma or infection
> - Neoplasm of effect of chemotherapy
> - Karyotype abnormalities (e.g., Klinefelter's syndrome)
> - Hemosiderosis
> - Mumps and severe epididymo-orchitis are the main inflammatory causes.

Obstructive male infertility

Obstruction can occur at any level of the male reproductive tract, from the rete testis and the epididymis to the vas deferens. Obstruction can be due to congenital, inflammatory, or iatrogenic causes.

Congenital absence of the vas deferens is associated with carriers of cystic fibrosis (10% of cases), thus pre-IVF screening for carrier status should be carried out.

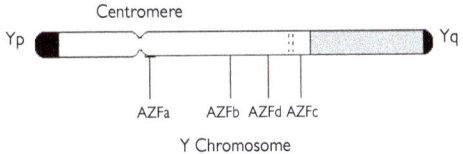

Figure 13.1 The Y chromosome.

Varicocele

A *varicocele* is the presence of abnormally tortuous veins of the pampiniform plexus within the spermatic cord. It is more common on the left that on the right because of the direct insertion of the spermatic vein into the left renal vein.

It occurs in both fertile and infertile males, but there appears to be a higher incidence in males with abnormal sperm parameters.

The impact of a varicocele on male fertility is controversial. It is argued by some that the varicocele causes an increase in local temperature in the testis that inhibits spermatogenesis. However, radiological and surgical correction is thought not to improve sperm function, so this line of management is not commonly used.

Autoimmune causes

Approximately 12% of men have antisperm antibodies. Incidence is significantly higher in men who have had trauma or surgery to the testis. The presence of the antibodies may lead to a decrease in sperm motility and may impede sperm binding to the zona pellucida, although low levels are not thought to have any significant effect.

Endocrine causes

This is a rare cause but will include hypogonadotropic hypogonadism and thyroid and adrenal disease. Hypogonadotropic hypogonadism may be idiopathic or due to Kallman syndrome, in which the hypogonadotropic hypogonadism is accompanied by anosmia.

Hyperprolactinemia in men may lead to impotence but has little effect on sperm production unless it leads to hypogonadism.

Environmental factors

Exposure to heat, chemicals, and ionizing irradiation can damage sperm production. The effects of environmental toxins and endocrine disruptors on male infertility are unclear, although epidemiological studies have shown a decline in sperm quality in the developed or industrial world.

Drugs

Both medicinal and recreational drugs can affect sperm function, as shown in Table 13.1.

Table 13.1 Effects of drugs on spermatogenesis

Drug	Effect on spermatogenesis	Effect on sperm function
Anabolic steroid	Yes	No
Antifungal	Yes	No
Sulfasalazine	Yes	No
Corticosteroids	Yes	No
Alcohol	Yes	Yes
Cigarettes	Yes	Yes
Marijuana	Yes	Yes
Opiates	Yes	Yes
Chemotherapy drug	Permanent sterility	

Investigation of the male

Semen analysis
The large biological variability seen in the quality of sperm in repeated tests on the same individual limits the reproducibility of semen analysis as a diagnostic test. Table 13.2 shows the accepted value for a semen analysis.

Many other tests of semen quality have been devised. These include biochemical analysis of the seminal fluid and detection of antisperm antibodies. Biochemical analysis of the seminal fluid can provide information about the prostate, seminal vesicles, and epididymis.

The detection of antisperm antibodies using immunobeads or the mixed antibody reaction (MAR) test is still in the WHO criteria; an MAR test of <50% sperm with adherent particles is described as normal.

Sperm function tests
Routine semen analysis gives an indication of sperm function simply by the measure of normality or non-normality. Some tests (Table 13.3) have been derived to try and measure sperm function as would occur in vivo. They are of academic interest and not of clinical value.

Table 13.2 Normal and abnormal semen parameters

Semen characteristics	Normal	Borderline	Pathological
Volume (mL)	2.0–6.0	1.5–2.0	<1.5
Sperm concentration (million/mL)	20–250	10–20	<10
Total sperm count (million/ejaculate)	>80	20–80	<20
Motility (0.5–2 hr after ejaculate)	>50	35–49	<35
Progression at 37°C (0–4)	3 or 4	2	<2
Vitality (% live)	≥75	50–74	<50
Morphology (/100 sperm)			
Head defects	<35	35–59	>60
Midpiece defects	≤20	21–25	>25
Tail defects	≤20	21–25	>25

Table 13.3 Sperm function tests

Hypo-osmotic swelling test
Test for sperm nuclear maturity
Measure of acrosome status
Acrosome reaction and acrosin activity
Hamster zona-free oocyte penetration
Human sperm–zona binding and penetration

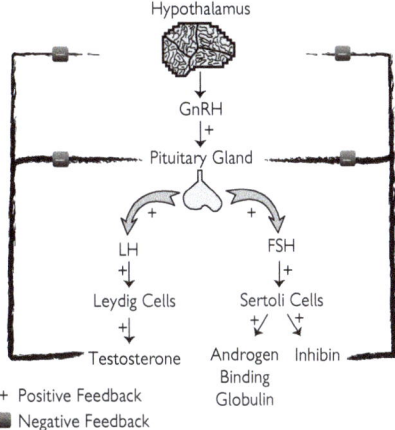

Figure 13.2 Normal gonadal–pituitary axis.

Hormonal analysis of the male

The objective of hormonal analysis is to determine whether the azoospermia is due to primary testicular failure or to an outflow obstruction. The normal gonadal–pituitary axis is shown in Fig. 13.2, and a flow diagram for investigation and diagnosis is shown in Fig. 13.3.

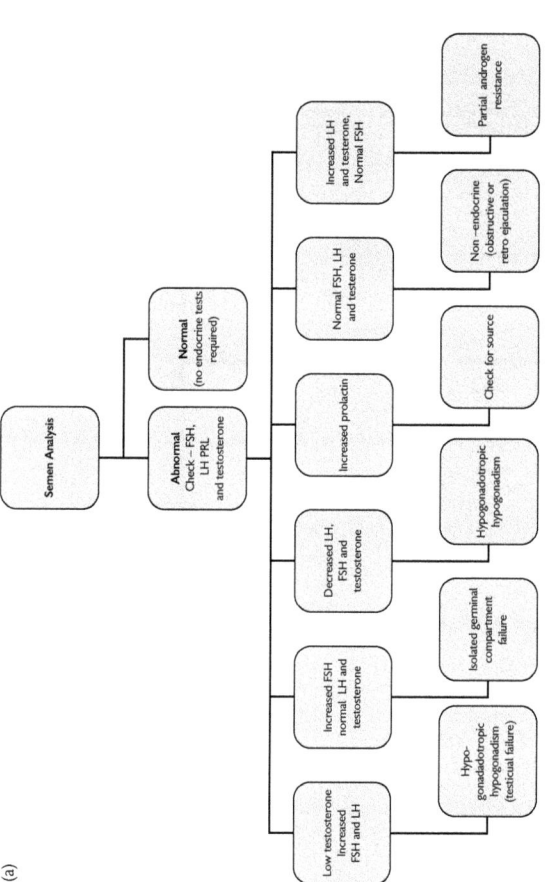

Figure 13.3 Hormonal investigations (a) of males and (b) of hypogonadotropic hypogonadism.

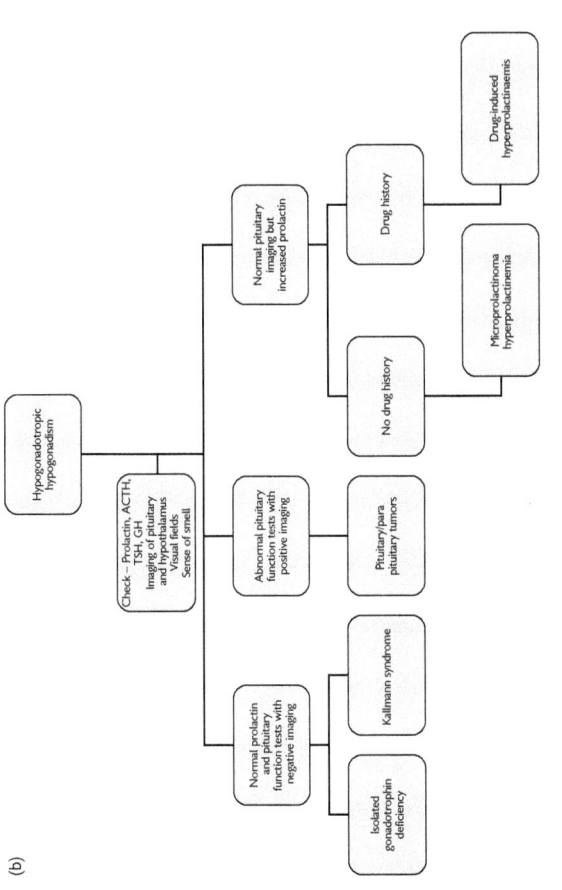

Figure 13.3 (Contd.)

Hypogonadotropic hypogonadism, often associated with Kallmann syndrome, has been successfully treated with pulsatile GnRH or hMG to restore spermatogenic drive and, hence, fertility.

Initiation of spermatogenesis can take several months.

Further reading and information

American Society for Reproductive Medicine: http://www.asrm.org/
European Society for Human Reproduction and Embryology: http://www.eshre.com/emc.asp

Chapter 14

Ovulation induction

Introduction *122*
Clomifene citrate *123*
Aromatase inhibitors *125*
Metformin *126*
Pulsatile gonadotropin-releasing hormone *127*
Gonadotropins *128*
Laparoscopic ovarian drilling (LOD) *133*
Further reading *133*

Introduction

Once the diagnosis of anovulation has been made and its cause determined (see Chapter 7), the starting treatment in that particular condition can also be determined.

The objective of ovulation induction is to restore the ovulatory state and reinstate fertility potential. Ideally, this should produce one ovulatory follicle and should not be confused with controlled ovarian stimulation for in vitro fertilization (IVF) or for intrauterine insemination (IUI), which is applied to already ovulating women with the aim of producing multiple ovulations.

The complications of ovulation induction are multiple pregnancies and ovarian hyperstimulation syndrome (OHSS). They are both caused by the induction of multiple follicular growth and are iatrogenic and largely preventable. Both can be avoided by expertise in recognition of the impending danger, action to be taken for their prevention, correct dosing, and adequate monitoring.

The number of large follicles induced influences the chances of a multiple pregnancy, whereas large numbers of intermediate- and small-sized follicles contribute to the incidence of OHSS.

In general, overweight and obesity are serious impeding factors in the attaining of a live birth following ovulation induction and in all other forms of treatment for infertility. Every attempt should be made to reduce the weight of overweight and frankly obese patients, through lifestyle changes involving dietary advice and exercise, before embarking on ovulation induction.

Obesity not only negatively influences the chances of conception but also increases the prevalence of spontaneous miscarriage. This is especially relevant for women with infertility associated with polycystic ovary syndrome (PCOS), as obesity exaggerates the deleterious effects of insulin resistance on fertility potential. A loss of just 5% or more of body weight is often enough to improve this situation.

Clomifene citrate

Indications

Clomifene citrate (CC) is the first-line treatment for women with absent or irregular ovulation associated with normal concentrations of endogenous estradiol and FSH (WHO Group 2, hypothalamic–pituitary dysfunction). A very large majority of these cases are associated with PCOS.

Mode of action

CC is an antiestrogenic compound closely resembling estrogen, which acts by blocking estrogen receptors, particularly in the hypothalamus, thereby signaling a lack of circulating estrogens and inducing a change in the pulsatile release of GnRH. This induces a discharge of FSH from the anterior pituitary and is often enough to reset the cycle of events leading to ovulation into motion.

Dose

CC (50 mg tablets) is given orally in a dose of 50–150 mg/day for 5 days from day 2, 3, 4, or 5 of a spontaneous or induced bleeding. The starting day of treatment does not seem to influence the results.

The recommended dose for the first cycle of treatment is 50 mg/day. If ovulation is achieved, there is no need to increase the dose in subsequent cycles.

If there is no response, i.e., no evidence of ovulation, the dose may be increased in increments of 50 mg in subsequent cycles until ovulation is achieved. An ovulatory response is reportedly achieved by 46% on 50 mg/day, a further 21% respond to 100 mg, and another 8% to 150 mg.

Doses >150 mg/day do not seem to confer any significant increase in either ovulation or pregnancy rates.

Results

The ovulation rate is 75%; pregnancy rate, 35%; live birth rate, 28–30%; miscarriage rate, 20%; twin pregnancy rate, 8–13%; and singleton live birth rate, 22%.

"Clomifene failure" may be due to a failure to respond with ovulation to maximal doses (clomifene resistance) or a failure to conceive following six ovulatory cycles.

Factors affecting results

Clomifene resistance is more likely to occur in patients who are obese, insulin resistant, and hyperandrogenic. A failure to conceive despite achieving ovulation may be due to the antiestrogen effects of CC, suppression of cervical mucus, and/or suppression of endometrial development (<7 mm thickness at mid-cycle). These effects are idiosyncratic, occur in ~15% of patients receiving CC, recur in repeated cycles, and are neither dose dependent nor improved by adding estrogen therapy.

IUI can overcome suppression of the cervical mucus, but endometrial suppression should preclude further attempts at treatment with CC, and low-dose FSH may be offered. Persistently high serum concentrations of LH are also thought to reduce the chances of pregnancy.

Duration of treatment

Of the pregnancies induced by CC, 75% occur in the first three cycles of treatment. Best practice is not to exceed 6 months of treatment.

There is little advantage to be gained by using a dose of >150 mg/day if this fails to produce ovulation. In this case, metformin added to CC or low-dose gonadotropins may be offered.

If three ovulatory cycles fail to yield a pregnancy, the couple should be referred to a reproductive endocrinologist for IVF.

Monitoring

CC is often administered without any monitoring of the treatment cycle. This is not good practice, as it is important to know whether ovulation has been achieved and whether endometrial development is normal.

A vaginal ultrasound examination on day 12–14 of a treatment cycle should suffice, as the number and size of developing follicles and endometrial thickness can be visualized easily.

Knowledge of the response to CC regarding follicular and endometrial development may save many months of superfluous treatment with an insufficient dose or in the presence of endometrial suppression.

Adjuvants for treatment with CC

An ovulation-triggering dose of hCG (5000–10,000 IU) when a follicle of 19–24 mm is demonstrated is only theoretically warranted when ovulation is not forthcoming in the presence of a leading follicle of this size because of the absence of an LH surge.

However, although the routine administration of hCG at mid-cycle seems to add little to the improvement of pregnancy rates, it is useful as an aid in the timing of IUI or intercourse.

Dexamethasone (0.5 mg daily at night) as an addition to CC treatment is probably best reserved for women who have evidence of an adrenal source of hyperandrogenism, such as late-onset congenital adrenal hyperplasia.

The possible pretreatment or addition of metformin to treatment with CC is discussed in a later section in this chapter.

Side effects

Adverse effects of clomifene are not common but include hot flashes, headache, ovarian hyperstimulation, abdominal distension, and visual disturbances. Visual disturbances warrant stopping clomifene therapy and proceeding to low-dose FSH stimulation.

Aromatase inhibitors

Although widely used for the treatment of postmenopausal women with advanced breast cancer, the use of aromatase inhibitors for induction of ovulation is still experimental and has not yet been fully sanctioned by the international community. However, several large trials have offered reassuring results.

The use of aromatase inhibitors for ovulation induction is briefly described here, as pending reassuring data on the outcome of pregnancies, it is believed that their use for ovulation induction has some advantages over CC as first-line treatment for WHO Group 2 anovulatory women.

Aromatase inhibitors (Letrozal 2.5–5 mg/day) are potent suppressors of estrogen synthesis, blocking the action of the enzyme aromatase. This converts androgens to estrogens, temporarily releasing the hypothalamus from the negative feedback effect of estrogen, thus inducing an increased discharge of FSH.

In contrast to CC, aromatase inhibitors have no effect on estrogen receptors and thus no deleterious effect on cervical mucus, endometrium, and the hypothalamic negative feedback mechanism. The half-life of the aromatase inhibitors is ~2 days, much shorter than that of CC.

Preliminary small trials have demonstrated the theoretical advantages of aromatase inhibitors over CC, the lack of an antiestrogen effect on endometrium and less multiple follicle development, while being equally efficient at induction of ovulation.

Large RCTs are awaited to confirm these preliminary results.

Metformin

Metformin is prescribed to reduce insulin and androgen concentrations and to treat anovulation associated with PCOS. Metformin is an oral biguanide that is well established for the treatment of hyperglycemia; it does not cause hypoglycemia in normoglycemic subjects.

Although there is some conflicting evidence regarding the usefulness of metformin and it is not currently licensed for the management of PCOS, it is being widely prescribed for this.

Indications

For restoration of ovulation for women with PCOS, metformin may be given alone or as pretreatment and co-treatment with CC. Proof of insulin resistance is not a prerequisite for treatment: first, this is difficult to assess accurately, and second, it does seem to predict the success of treatment.

Mode of action

Metformin is an insulin sensitizer that reduces insulin resistance and insulin secretion, followed by a reduction of ovarian androgen production. A direct action of metformin on ovarian theca cells also reduces androgen production.

Dose

- Metformin is taken orally in doses of 1500–2500 mg daily.

Side effects

About 15–20% of patients may suffer gastrointestinal side effects, some of which may be lessened by a graduated starting dose.

Metformin alone

Metformin is capable of improving menstrual frequency and restoring ovulation in patients who have olig- or /anovulation and PCOS, although less effectively than clomifene alone.

However, for obese patients (BMI >30), metformin (1700 mg/day) was no better than placebo in improving menstrual function, whereas weight loss was effective. Most studies have shown no increase or only a modest increase in pregnancy rates.

Metformin + CC

Some initial collected reports suggested that the combination of pretreatment and co-treatment of metformin with CC is significantly more successful at inducing ovulation and pregnancy than the use of metformin alone or CC alone.

However, in previously untreated women with PCOS, no superiority of the combination of CC and metformin over CC alone was demonstrated in a large multicenter study from the Netherlands, nor in a large American study that also demonstrated no superiority of the combination over metformin alone.

Metformin added to CC therapy in CC-resistant patients and CC administered to those who failed to ovulate on metformin alone will achieve ovulation and pregnancy in some women and may be tried before turning to the more costly FSH therapy.

Metformin in IVF

Two well-controlled studies have shown superiority in pregnancy rates in nonobese women with PCOS, compared with placebo, when metformin was started either 6 weeks before or at the start of a GnRH agonist long protocol.

Metformin in pregnancy

Metformin appears to be safe when continued into pregnancy, as no increase in congenital abnormalities, teratogenicity, or adverse effects on infant development have been recorded.

There is conflicting evidence regarding the ability of metformin to reduce the high miscarriage rate that usually occurs among PCOS patients to levels seen in the normal population.

Whether metformin should be continued into the pregnancy is still disputed.

Pulsatile gonadotropin-releasing hormone (gonadorelin)

Pulsatile GnRH therapy is the classical treatment of anovulation associated with hypogonadotropic hypogonadism (WHO Group 2) and can be regarded as pure replacement therapy to restore the function of the anterior pituitary in discharging FSH and LH. It can be used as an alternative to gonadotropin therapy with both FSH and LH activity. Because of its inconvenience, expense, and low pregnancy rate compared with that of other forms of treatment, this therapy is no longer used in practice.

GnRH is administered through an infusion pump, very similar to an insulin pump, either subcutaneously (SC) or intravenously (IV).

The dose is a bolus of 15–20 mcg SC or 5–10 mcg IV every 60–90 minutes. Very occasionally, thrombophlebitis is experienced at the site of the indwelling catheter when the IV route is used.

Pulsatile GnRH is very effective treatment for idiopathic hypogonadotropic hypogonadism, Kallmann's syndrome, and low-weight-related amenorrhea, producing pregnancy rates well in excess of 80%.

Following ovulation, the pump must be continued into the luteal phase. If stopped following ovulation, then luteal phase support is required.

For the treatment of WHO Group 1 anovulation, compared with gonadotropin treatment, GnRH has the advantage of producing a monofollicular ovulation in the vast majority of cycles and a consequent low rate of multiple pregnancy.

The disadvantage of pulsatile GnRH therapy is the inconvenience of wearing the pump and accoutrements; this has limited patient acceptability.

Gonadotropins

Gonadotropin preparations containing FSH provide an exogenous source for the direct stimulus of follicular development in anovulatory women. hCG mimics the action of the LH surge and is used to trigger ovulation once a stimulated follicle(s) has reached a stage of development when ovulation can be induced.

The aim of ovulation induction with gonadotropins is to produce, ideally, one ovulatory follicle, so avoiding the complications of multiple follicular development, OHSS and multiple pregnancies.

Because of these significant and life-threatening side effects, gonadotropins should only be administered by those with extreme training and experience.

FSH-containing preparations

These preparations may be derived from human menopausal urine from which either FSH or FSH + LH are extracted and purified or from the use of recombinant DNA technology to produce recombinant human FSH. Large RCTs and meta-analyses comparing the use of urinary-derived and recombinant preparations for ovulation induction have shown no significant differences regarding ovulation and pregnancy rates, miscarriage, hyperstimulation, or multiple pregnancy rates.

As far as the outcome of gonadotropin ovulation induction therapy is concerned, no clear clinical superiority has been demonstrated between preparations containing LH (hMG) and those containing FSH alone.

Only for women with hypogonadotropic hypogonadism is LH an essential component to ensure efficient and successful ovulation induction.

Delivery systems

Both recombinant FSH preparations (follitropin α and follitropin β) are now available as ready-to-use preparations in a pen injection device that comes either preloaded containing 300, 450, or 900 IU (follitropin α, Gonal-F®, Merk, Serono) or in cartridges for loading containing 300, 600, or 900 IU recombinant FSH (follitropin β, follestim).

With pen devices, the FSH dose can be accurately titrated and individualized for each patient for SC injection and is more user-friendly.

Urinary products containing purified FSH or FSH with LH are sold as lyophilized powders that are mixed with sterile water after injection.

Indications

For ovulation induction, gonadotropin therapy is indicated for hypogonadotropic hypogonadism (WHO Group I) if preferred to pulsatile GnRH therapy. For women with hypogonadotropic hypogonadism, it is essential to use an LH-containing preparation or to add recombinant LH to FSH in order to ensure efficient ovulation induction.

More commonly, gonadotropins are used for those with WHO Group II anovulation who either did not respond to CC or failed to conceive following up to six ovulatory cycles on CC.

Treatment protocol

Conventional, regular protocol

Gonadotropin treatment is started on day 3 of menstruation, natural or induced, when the ovary is quiescent and the endometrium thin. Using a regular, conventional protocol, the initial dose in the first cycle of treatment has usually been one ampoule a day of hMG (75 IU FSH + 75 IU LH) or 75 IU of FSH with incremental dose rises of one ampoule of hMG or 50–75 IU of FSH every 5–7 days if an inadequate response (no follicle >9 mm) is recorded on ultrasound examination.

Ovulation is triggered with a single intramuscular (IM) injection of 5000–10,000 IU of hCG when 1–3 follicles reach a diameter of at least 17 mm. The starting dose in subsequent cycles could be adjusted according to the response in the previous cycle.

The conventional protocol has been largely abandoned, certainly for women with Group II anovulation, as it produced multiple pregnancy rates of 34% and severe OHSS in 4.6%. As these figures are unacceptable today, a chronic low-dose protocol has been devised and applied.

Low-dose step-up protocol

The aim of the chronic low-dose step-up protocol is to obtain the ovulation of a single follicle. Unlike the conventional protocol, the low-dose protocol has a dose of gonadotropin that is not supraphysiological but reaches the threshold for a follicular response without exceeding it, thereby producing monofollicular rather than multifollicular ovulation. This practically eliminates the occurrence of OHSS and reduces multiple pregnancies to an acceptable rate.

The chronic low-dose regimen (illustrated in Fig. 14.1) has a small starting dose in the first cycle of treatment of 50–75 IU of FSH, which remains unchanged for 14 days. If this does not produce the criteria for hCG administration, a small incremental dose rise of 25–37.5 IU is used every 7 days until follicular development is initiated.

The dose that initiates follicular development (at least one follicle >10 mm) is continued until the criteria for giving hCG are attained. hCG should not be given if ≥3 follicles >16 mm diameter are seen.

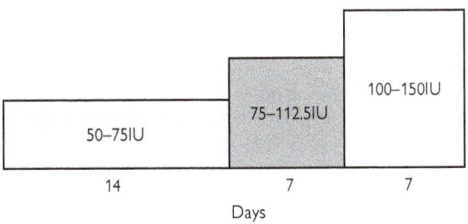

Figure 14.1 The chronic low-dose step-up regimen for the administration of gonadotropin.

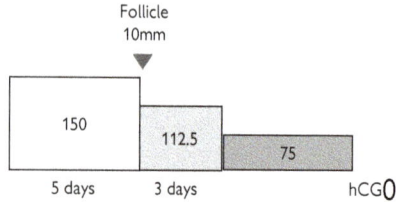

Figure 14.2 The step-down protocol.

Use of a starting dose of 75 IU FSH ensures that ~90% of women will not require any dose adjustment, whereas starting with 50 IU of FSH requires a dose adjustment in ~50% of women.

Step-down protocol
On the basis of physiological principles concerning concentrations of FSH in a natural ovulatory cycle, a step-down protocol has been suggested, starting with 150 IU of FSH for 5 days, raising the dose by 37.5 IU every 3 days if necessary, until a follicle of 10 mm is obtained (Fig. 14.2). The daily dose is then reduced by 37.5 IU every 3 days until the criteria for giving hCG are reached.

However, although pregnancy rates are similar and FSH is given for a shorter duration with step-down, the low-dose step-up has a lower rate of overstimulation, double the rate of monofollicular ovulation, and a higher ovulation rate and is, therefore, preferred by most.

Monitoring

The timing of a possible increase in dose and the timing of hCG administration are the essence of efficient ovulation induction and avoidance of OHSS and multiple pregnancies with gonadotropin therapy. Accurate monitoring of follicular development by transvaginal ultrasound examination of the ovaries and endometrial thickness is the key factor.

Most practices also estimate serum estradiol concentrations on the same day as the ultrasound examination, but some reserve these examinations only for women at high risk for OHSS. The first examination is usually performed on day 5 of stimulation.

Once an emerging follicle of ≥10 mm diameter is seen, the daily effective dose used to achieve this should not be changed and further examinations performed every 2–3 days following. As a rough rule of thumb, an emerging leading follicle will grow at a rate of 2 mm/day on the daily effective dose.

The criteria for administering hCG in a dose of 5000–10,000 IU are 1–2 follicles of ≥18 mm. If hCG is given when >2 follicles of this size are attained, the risk of a multiple pregnancy is increased considerably.

Ovarian hyperstimulation syndrome (OHSS)

OHSS is a serious complication of ovulation induction caused by over-stimulating the ovaries with gonadotropins followed by hCG to trigger ovulation. It is an iatrogenic condition that is largely preventable and often foreseeable.

Women at greatest risk of developing OHSS are young and lean and have polycystic ovaries. The occurrence of OHSS in a previous cycle is also a predisposing factor that should induce watchfulness.

Prevention of OHSS

If hCG is withheld, OHSS typically will not occur.

For patients with risk factors for OHSS, a small starting dose and small incremental dose rises if needed in a chronic low-dose protocol will prevent OHSS.

If the danger of OHSS looks imminent during ovulation stimulation (a large number of developing follicles, rapidly rising estradiol concentrations, very high estradiol concentrations >1500 pg/mL or 5500 pmol/mL), hCG should be withheld. It is better to lose a cycle than take the risk of severe OHSS.

Alternatively, coasting may be employed by withdrawing gonadotropin therapy and checking the number and size of follicles and estradiol concentrations daily thereafter until hCG can safely be given, when coasting has caused a regression in the number of follicles and a decrease in estradiol concentrations. Coasting has only proved to be effective if the interval between stopping gonadotropins and giving hCG does not exceed 3 days.

A less popular recourse for action if overstimulation occurs during ovulation induction entails follicle puncture, oocyte retrieval, and IVF, so-called rescue IVF.

Giving one injection of a GnRH agonist to trigger a release of endogenous LH in place of hCG has met with some success in ovulation induction facing possible OHSS. The shorter half-life of a GnRH agonist than that of hCG is thought to be the important difference between the two.

For a similar reason, recombinant LH can be used instead of hCG.

Prevention of multiple pregnancies

During ovulation induction, the risk of a multiple pregnancy increases when hCG is given when >2 large follicles have developed. The hCG injection may be withheld in this situation. Using a strict chronic low-dose protocol, this should be a rare occurrence.

Results

Using a conventional protocol for WHO Group I and Group II anovulation, a collection of results published in 1990 indicated a pregnancy rate of 46% but a multiple pregnancy rate of 34% and a prevalence of 4.6% of severe OHSS. Following the inception of a chronic low-dose protocol, while the pregnancy rate is similar, multiple pregnancy occurs in <6%, and OHSS has been virtually eliminated (Table 14.1).

Table 14.1 Results of treatment with chronic low-dose gonadotropin

No. of patients	841
No. of cycles	1556
Pregnancies (% patients)	320 (38%)
Fecundity/cycle	20%
Uniovulation	70%
OHSS	0.14%
Multiple pregnancies	5.7%

Laparoscopic ovarian drilling (LOD)

The original treatment of PCOS instigated by Stein and Leventhal was bilateral wedge resection of the ovaries. Although this procedure produced restoration of ovulation in a high proportion of women and induced pregnancy, it was abandoned because of a high prevalence of pelvic adhesion formation.

The principle of operational treatment (presumably a reduction in ovarian mass) has been largely replaced by LOD.

On laparoscopy, 4–10 punctures with a depth of 2–4 mm are made in the cortex of each ovary. Fewer than four punctures are ineffective and >10 create too much damage to the ovary. Using bipolar or unipolar electrocautery, 40W for 4 seconds for each puncture is a good rule of thumb. Laser can also be used, but electrocautery is reported to produce better results with less adhesion formation.

An ovulation rate of 84% and a pregnancy rate of 56% were experienced within 1 year of LOD in the first collection of reports. In a single-center study of long-term follow-up, 49% of patients conceived spontaneously within a year and a further 38% conceived 1–9 years after LOD. The cumulative conception rate after 30 months was 75%.

If no ovulation results within 2–3 months of LOD, administration of CC will induce ovulation in many who were previously resistant to CC and, if this is not successful, a low-dose FSH protocol can be applied. The addition of CC or FSH following drilling considerably increases pregnancy rates.

Women with PCOS of normal weight and with high LH concentrations are those most likely to ovulate and conceive following treatment by LOD.

The advantage of LOD for ovulation induction in women with PCOS is that almost invariably it will produce a monofollicular ovulation and therefore a very low rate of multiple pregnancies and no OHSS. In addition, the miscarriage rate following LOD (14%) is lower than that usually experienced with other forms of ovulation induction for PCOS.

Potential disadvantages include adhesion formation and destruction of the ovary with potential loss of ovarian follicular reserve.

Further reading

Hamilton-Fairly O, Frank S (1990). Common problems in induction of ovulation. *Ballieres Clin Obstet Gynaecol* 4:609–625.

Kousta E, White DM, Franks S (1997). Modern use of clomiphene citrate in induction of ovulation. *Hum Reprod Update* 3:359–365.

Moll E, Bossyuyt PM, Korevaar JC, Lambalk CB, van der Veen F (2006). Effect of clomiphene citrate plus metformin and clomiphene citrate plus placebo on induction of ovulation in women with newly diagnosed polycystic ovary syndrome: a randomized double blind clinical trial. *BMJ* 332:1485.

Chapter 15

Tubal and uterine disorders

Introduction *136*
Tubal disorders *137*
Surgery to the fallopian tube *139*
Uterine disorders *140*

Introduction

Normal conception requires a fertile sperm and an egg to come together and a receptive endometrium to allow the resulting embryo to implant. Tubal damage underlies infertility in ~15% of couples. In some of these couples, it may be that the woman has previously undergone a tubal sterilization procedure for conception but wish to have this reversed.

Whereas tubal occlusion or damage is a relatively clear-cut cause of infertility, the presence of uterine fibroids is less absolute as an explanation for their infertility.

This is also the case for intrauterine adhesion and congenital abnormalities of the uterus.

Tubal disorders

Any damage to the fallopian tube can prevent the sperm from reaching the oocyte or the embryo from reaching the uterine cavity, leading to infertility and tubal ectopic pregnancy.

The fallopian tube is more than a simple tube. It has cilia that assist in transport, and it facilitates capacitation of the sperm and fertilization and the early development of the zygote and embryo. Therefore, the fallopian tube may maintain its patency but lose the ability to promote these other functions.

Anatomy

The fallopian tubes are seromuscular paired tubular organs that run medially from the ovaries to the cornua of the uterus. The fallopian tubes are situated toward the upper margins of the broad ligament.

The tubes connect the endometrial cavity in the uterus with the peritoneal cavity toward the ovaries on each side. The tubes average 10 cm in length (range, 7–14 cm).

The tubes can be divided into four parts (proximally at the endometrial cavity to their distal portion near the ovary):
- The intramural or interstitial portion (from the endometrial cavity, through the uterine wall, and to the uterine cornua)
- The isthmus (the proximal third of the fallopian tubes outside the uterine wall)
- The ampulla (the distal two-thirds of the fallopian tubes outside the uterine wall)
- The infundibulum, the funnel-shaped opening to the peritoneal cavity

The fimbria are finger-like extensions from the margins of the infundibulum toward the ovaries on each side. The intraluminal diameter varies and increases from 0.1 mm in the intramural portion to 1 cm in the ampullary portion of the tubes.

The fallopian tubes receive their blood supply from the tubal branches of the uterine arteries and from small branches of the ovarian arteries. The fallopian tubes receive sensory, autonomic, and vasomotor nerve fibers from the ovarian and inferior hypogastric plexi.

Pathophysiology

The main causes of tubal disease are either pelvic inflammatory disease (PID) or iatrogenic causes. PID commonly causes tubal blockage, either proximally at the site of insertion into the uterus or distally at the fimbrial end. Less commonly, a midtubal segment may become occluded.

Blockage at two points results in a hydrosalpinx, because the continued secretions of the tubal mucosa have no drainage into the peritoneal or uterine cavities. As the hydrosalpinx enlarges, the tubal muscularis thins. The secretory and ciliary properties of the endosalpinx are eventually disrupted.

The probability of pregnancy after repair of hydrosalpinges with a diameter of >3 cm is very poor.

The pathophysiology after tubal sterilization depends on the method used. The method most commonly used in the United States often causes great damage to the fallopian tube and therefore the procedure is not easily reversed. Electrocautery of a segment or segments of the fallopian tube occludes the lumen and causes more damage to the surrounding tissues than placement of a ring or a clip over the mid-portion of the tube or surgical interruption of the tube.

Increasing the amount of damage to the fallopian tube may increase the success of the sterilization procedure, but it decreases the chance of achieving subsequent successful reconstruction. The length of a tube after a reconstructive procedure correlates with success in terms of achieving pregnancy. Patients with tubes >5 cm after reconstruction have better outcomes than patients whose tubes measure ≤3 cm.

Any inflammatory condition in the pelvis, such as endometriosis or the sequelae of pelvic or abdominal surgery, may cause adhesions, tubal blockage, or injury to the tubal mucosa and/or muscularis, resulting in tubal damage and dysfunction. In some women, cornual polyps may develop in the fallopian tube, causing a blockage that may be reversible by resection of the polyp.

Salpingitis isthmica nodosa

Proximal tubal disease can also be caused by salpingitis isthmica nodosa. It is commonly diagnosed when firm nodules are found on the fallopian tubes. The diagnosis is confirmed by histopathology.

The hallmark of salpingitis isthmica nodosa is the presence of diverticula or outpouchings of the tubal epithelium, which are surrounded by hypertrophied smooth muscle.

The diagnosis can only be confirmed by histology. It can be suspected by hysterosalpingography if proximal obstruction is present or by a stippled appearance indicating contrast medium in the diverticular projections. The cause of salpingitis isthmica nodosa is not known.

Salpingitis isthmica nodosa is found in 0.6–11% of healthy fertile women and is almost always bilateral.

Surgery to the fallopian tube

Any surgery to the fallopian tube that is designed to restore or improve fertility should involve microsurgical techniques. These techniques are more commonly used at open surgery but are increasingly being performed through endoscopic surgery.

Microsurgical technique is a delicate surgical style that emphasizes the use of magnification, fine atraumatic instrumentation, microsuturing, continuous irrigation to prevent desiccation, and pinpoint hemostasis.

The goals are to remove pathology, restore normal anatomy and regain function with minimal damage to adjacent normal tissue. This is achieved by minimizing inflammation and preventing adhesion formation.

Intramural or interstitial obstruction

This is one of the more challenging surgeries to perform, as it often involves tubal reimplantation after the resection of cornual polyps. In some cases, patency can be restored by hysteroscopic or radiological cannulation.

The tubal ostia are visualized in the endometrial cavity with the hysteroscope or under radiological control. A small wire is inserted through the os into the intramural portion of the tube, and a small catheter is threaded over the wire.

Patency can be confirmed when dye introduced through the small catheter in the intramural portion of the tube is visualized extruding through the fimbria via laparoscopy or radiologically.

Isthmic and mid-portion occlusion (including reversal of sterilization)

Isthmic occlusion can be repaired by performing an isthmic–cornual or an isthmic–isthmic anastomosis, as appropriate.

The damaged portion of the tube is transected perpendicular to the axis of the tube. The occluded portion of the tube is resected 2 mm at a time, initially proximally and subsequently distally, until the tubal lumen is visualized.

Proximal patency is confirmed using retrograde methylene blue through a cannula in the uterine cavity. Distal patency is confirmed by threading a piece of thin suture material from the fimbrial end toward the area of anastomosis.

An anchoring suture is placed in the proximal and distal mesosalpinx (isthmic–isthmic repair) or from the cornu proximally to the mesosalpinx distally (cornual–isthmic repair) to bring the two portions of the tube being reanastomosed in proximity. Four interrupted sutures are placed at the 12-, 3-, 6- and 9-o'clock positions, parallel to the axis of the tube, first within the muscularis (using a 8.0 non-absorbable suture, e.g. prolene) and subsequently on the serosa (6.0 prolene), to bring together the proximal and distal portions of the tube.

For reversal of sterilization, depending on the patient's age, pregnancy rates should be in the order of 80% in the first year.[1]

---

1 Boeckx W, Gordts S, Buysse K, Brosens I (1986). Reversibility after female sterilization. *Br J Obstet Gynaecol* 93:839–842.

Occlusion of the distal portion of the fallopian tube
This usually involves a fimbroplasty. Proximal patency of the tube should be confirmed with a preoperative hysterosalpingogram.

Filling the fallopian tube with dilute dye at the time of surgery (via a cannula in the uterine cavity) facilitates identification of the entrance point in the distal, peritoneal surface of the tube that opens into the tubal lumen. The entrance point, which should be relatively avascular, is then opened using scissors, needle point diathermy or laser. The fimbria are then retracted using either sutures or thermal damage to the peritoneal surface of the tube proximal to the fimbria.

Results of surgery
A case series study reported that 27%, 47%, and 53% of women with proximal tubal blockage who had microsurgical tubocornual anastomosis achieved a live birth within 1, 2, and 3.5 years of surgery, respectively.

A review of nine other case series studies reported that ~50% of women with proximal tubal blockage who had microsurgical tubocornual anastomosis achieved a term pregnancy, but it did not specify the time period upon which this figure was based.

Surgery is more effective in women with milder pelvic disease (stage I, 67%; stage II, 41%; stage III, 12%; and stage IV, 0%).

Uterine disorders

Submucous leiomyomata, congenital uterine abnormalities, endometrial polyps, and intrauterine adhesions are all potential causes of infertility.

The presence of a fibroid that distorts the fallopian tubes will lead to tubal infertility. Distortion of the uterine cavity, by a fibroid, a septum, or a congenitally misshaped uterus, can lead to implantation failure and/or recurrent miscarriage.

Recent evidence has also suggested that intramural fibroids inhibit implantation to a lesser degree. Removal of these intramural fibroids may result in an increased fertility level.

Excessive uterine curettage, e.g., after a miscarriage, especially in the presence of infection, can lead to distortion of the strata basalis endometrium. Intrauterine scarification and synechiae develop as a result, and this is known as Asherman's syndrome.

Uterine fibroids
The incidence of myoma in women with infertility without any other cause for their infertility is estimated to be ~2%.

Submuscosal fibroids may be removed hysteroscopically, with intramural and subserosal fibroids being removed either at open surgery or, if <9 cm in size, laparoscopically.

Microsurgical techniques described earlier in this chapter should be used and, if available, antiadhesion devices used following surgery for intramural and subserosal fibroids.

Chapter 16

Medical and surgical management of endometriosis

Introduction *142*
Examination and investigations *143*
Endometriosis-associated infertility *144*
Surgical treatment of endometriosis *145*
Principles of surgery for infertility patients with endometriosis *147*
Medical treatment *148*
Further reading and information *150*

Introduction

Endometriosis is characterized by the presence of endometrial tissue (glandular and stromal tissue) in areas outside the uterus. For decades it has been considered to be the result of the implantation of retrograde menstruated endometrial cells (Sampson's theory) or as metaplasia induced by menstrual debris or as lymphatic spread.

It occurs most frequently in the pelvic organs and peritoneum and is prevalent in 2.5–3.3% of women of reproductive age. Endometriosis is a surgical diagnosis.

In a hospital-based population, however, the prevalence of endometriosis will vary depending on the type of the population being studied; e.g., it is seen more frequently among women being investigated for infertility (up to 50%) than among those undergoing sterilization (6%).

The incidence of endometriosis among those women being investigated for chronic pelvic pain is also high, reaching approximately 50% in some studies. A more realistic estimate is that it affects approximately 10% of reproductive-age females.

Examination and investigations

The symptoms associated with endometriosis, principally dysmenorrhea, dyspareunia, and pelvic pain, are common. Establishing the diagnosis can be difficult because the presentation is so variable and there is considerable overlap with other conditions, such as irritable bowel syndrome and pelvic inflammatory disease (PID). As a result, there is often delay between symptom onset and surgical diagnosis.

Endometriosis may present with any combination of the following: secondary dysmenorrhea, deep dyspareunia, pelvic pain, infertility, or a pelvic mass. However, the predictive value of any one symptom or set of symptoms remains uncertain. Furthermore, endometriosis is often found coincidentally in asymptomatic women.

Laparoscopy is still regarded as the gold-standard diagnostic test in looking for evidence of all types and stages of endometriosis. However, diagnostic laparoscopy is associated with a 0.06% risk of major complications (e.g., bowel perforation); this risk is increased to 1.3% in operative laparoscopy.

The use of transvaginal ultrasound may be helpful in diagnosis, particularly to detect ovarian endometriomas. A systematic review on the accuracy of ultrasound identified seven relevant studies, all using transvaginal ultrasound (TU/S) to diagnose endometriomas. The positive likelihood ratios ranged from 7.6 to 29.8, and the negative likelihood ratios ranged from 0.12 to 0.4. TU/S, therefore, appears to be a useful test both to make and to exclude the diagnosis of an ovarian endometrioma.

It is incomplete, however, for identifying peritoneal endometriosis. Other imaging modalities include CT and MRI, and they are also limited.

Serum CA-125 testing has limited value as a screening test for endometriosis. The performance of CA-125 measurement was assessed in a meta-analysis: 23 studies had investigated serum CA-125 levels in women with surgically confirmed endometriosis. The test's performance in diagnosing all disease stages was limited: the estimated sensitivity was only 28% for a specificity of 90% (corresponding likelihood ratio of a raised level was 2.8). The test's performance for moderate to severe endometriosis was better: for a specificity of 89%, the sensitivity was 47% (corresponding likelihood ratio of a raised level was 4.3).

The routine use of serum CA-125 testing, particularly in subfertile patients, may be justified to identify a subgroup of women who are likely to benefit from early laparoscopy.

Thus CA-125 has limited value as a screening test as well as a diagnostic test. It may, however, serve as a useful marker for monitoring the effect of treatment once the diagnosis of endometriosis has been established, but again, its use has not been evaluated systematically.

The choice of treatment of endometriosis will depend on the woman's age, her fertility plans, previous treatment, the nature and severity of the symptoms, and the location and severity of disease.

Endometriosis-associated infertility

Arguments that support the hypothesis of a strong association, possibly a causal relationship, between the presence of endometriosis and subfertility include the following:
- An increased prevalence of endometriosis in subfertile women compared with that in women of proven fertility
- A trend toward a reduced monthly fecundity rate in infertile women with minimal to mild endometriosis compared with that in women with unexplained infertility
- A dose–effect relationship: a negative correlation between the revised American Society for Reproductive Medicine (ASRM) stage of endometriosis and the monthly fecundity rate and crude pregnancy rate
- A reduced number of oocytes, fertilization rate, implantation rate per embryo, and pregnancy rate after in vitro fertilization (IVF) in women with moderate to severe endometriosis compared with that in women with a normal pelvis
- An increased monthly fecundity rate and cumulative pregnancy rate after surgical removal of minimal to mild endometriosis

Surgical treatment of endometriosis

In most women with endometriosis, preservation of reproductive function is desirable. Therefore, the least invasive and least expensive approach that is effective should be used.

The goal of surgery is to excise, coagulate, or evaporate all visible endometriotic peritoneal lesions, endometriotic ovarian cysts, deep rectovaginal endometriosis, and associated adhesions and to restore normal anatomy.

Surgery should be performed by laparoscopy, as this affords the magnification and detail required to remove all lesions. It is also less invasive than laparotomy. For more severe disease, referral to a center specializing in endometriosis surgery may be required.

Cystic ovarian endometriosis

The physiopathology of cystic endometriosis is not entirely understood. It is postulated that many cases of cystic ovarian endometriosis may originate from invagination of superficial implants.

The management of ovarian cystic endometriosis (endometriomas) will depend to some extent on the size of the cyst. Small ovarian endometriomata (<3 cm diameter) can be aspirated and irrigated; their interior wall can be vaporized to destroy the mucosal lining of the cyst. Large (>3 cm in diameter) ovarian endometriomata should be aspirated, followed by incision and removal of the cyst wall from the ovarian cortex.

To prevent recurrence, the cyst wall of the endometrioma must be removed and normal ovarian tissue must be preserved (Table 16.1).

The use of the combined oral contraceptive (OC or GnRH agonist) prior to surgery may help to avoid confusion or inadvertent surgery on a corpus luteum. Postoperative OC use will reduce recurrence in the patient who does not want to conceive immediately.

Peritoneum endometriosis

Peritoneal implants can be ablated or excised. Excision results in a longer time to recurrence than ablation. However, ablation followed by GnRH agonist gives equivalent results.

Deep rectovaginal and rectosigmoidal endometriosis

Endometriosis can infiltrate the surrounding tissues, resulting in a sclerotic and inflammatory reaction that can translate clinically into nodularity,

Table 16.1 Removal versus ablation of emdometriomas*

Recurrence after coagulation or laser	Recurrence after cystectomy
18.4%	6.4%

*The results were from a systematic review of four comparative trials. Common odds ratio: 3.09 (95% CI 1.78–5.36).

Reprinted with permission from Vercellini P, Chapron C, De Giorgi O, et al. (2003). Coagulation or excision of ovarian endometriomas? *Am J Obstet Gynecol* 188: 606–610.

bowel stenosis, and ureteral obstruction. The most severe forms are rectovaginal endometriosis and endometriosis invading the rectum or the sigmoid. Three subtypes are described (Fig. 16.1):

- Type 1: large pelvic area of typical and sometimes some subtle endometriotic lesions surrounded by white sclerotic tissue
- Type 2: characterized by retraction of the bowel. Clinically, they are recognized by the obvious bowel retraction around a small typical lesion.
- Type 3: spherical endometriotic nodules in the rectovaginal septum. In their most typical manifestation, these lesions are felt as painful nodularities in the rectovaginal septum.

Type 3 lesions are the most severe lesions. They often spread laterally up and around the uterine artery, sometimes causing sclerosis around the ureter. Sclerosing endometriosis invading the sigmoid is similar to rectal endometriosis but is situated 10 cm above the rectovaginal septum. This is another form of deep endometriosis, which is a rare condition.

Surgery for deep endometriosis is unpredictably difficult, with the risk of a series of severe complications. Therefore, a preoperative ultrasound, contrast enema and IV pyelography are necessary in many cases, together with a full preoperative bowel preparation.

Surgery should be carefully planned. This planning comprises preoperative ureter stenting if gross ureteric distortion or hydronephrosis is present, together with the eventual collaboration of a urologist to perform ureter reanastomosis or repair, bladder suturing, or ureter re-implantation.

Preoperative planning often requires the collaboration of a colorectal surgeon, since surgery can unpredictably extend from a discoid excision with a muscularis defect, to resection of the rectum or sigmoid wall necessitating a suture, to a large transmural nodule requiring resection anastomosis if the defect is too large, or in the case of a combined rectal and sigmoid nodule that cannot be sutured, to a pouch anastomosis requiring mobilization of the left hemicolon.

Most women who have pain as a result of their endometriosis will also desire fertility. The result of fertility after surgery should be considered.

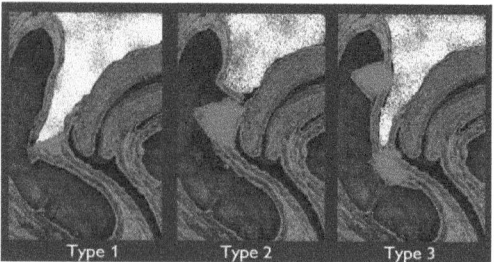

Figure 16.1 Deep rectovaginal or sigmoidal endometriosis.

Principles of surgery for infertility patients with endometriosis

Box 16.1 Principles of surgery for endometriosis in infertile patients

1. Women with minimal or mild endometriosis who undergo laparoscopy should be offered surgical ablation or resection of endometriosis plus laparoscopic adhesiolysis because this improves the chance of later pregnancy. The Endocan study was a large prospective randomized trial that compared diagnostic laparoscopy to ovarian laparoscopy in women with mild to moderate endometriosis. Ovulation therapy increased the pregnancy rate from approximately 18 years old to 30 years old over 9 months. While succeeding in improving fertility, the number headed to trail is 12. Most women with mild to moderate disease will have a greater chance of conceiving with assisted reproductive technologies (ART). If pain and infertility occur concurrently, the surgical treatment should be used.
2. Women with ovarian endometriomas should be offered laparoscopic cystectomy because this improves the chances of later pregnancy. However, there is concern that surgical intervention may diminish ovarian reserve.
3. Women with moderate or severe endometriosis should be offered surgical treatment or ART because it improves the chances of later pregnancy.
4. Postoperative medical treatment does not improve pregnancy rates in women with moderate to severe endometriosis and is not recommended.

Medical treatment

Because estrogen is known to stimulate the growth of endometriosis, hormonal therapy has been designed to suppress estrogen synthesis, thereby inducing atrophy of ectopic endometrial implants or interrupting the cycle of stimulation and bleeding. Implants of endometriosis react to gonadal steroid hormones in a manner that is similar but not identical to that of normally stimulated ectopic endometrium.

Ectopic endometrial tissue displays histological and biochemical differences from normal ectopic endometrium in characteristics such as glandular activity (proliferation, secretion), enzyme activity (aromatase 17-α-hydroxysteroid dehydrogenase), and steroid (estrogen, progestin, and androgen) hormone receptor levels.

Oral contraceptive pill

The treatment of endometriosis with continuous low-dose monophasic combination contraceptives (one pill per day for 6–12 months) has been shown to be effective in reducing dysmenorrhea and pelvic pain. In addition, the subsequent amenorrhea induced by oral contraceptives (OCs) could potentially reduce the amount of retrograde menstruation (one of the many risk factors proposed in the etiology of endometriosis), decreasing the risk of disease progression.

There is no convincing evidence that medical therapy with an OC offers definitive therapy. Instead, the endometrial implants survive the induced atrophy, with reactivation in most patients following termination of treatment.

There is no convincing evidence that cyclic use of combined OCs provide prophylaxis against the endometriosis. Estrogens in OCs may stimulate the proliferation of endometriosis. The reduced menstrual bleeding that often occurs in women taking OCs may be beneficial to women with prolonged, frequent menstrual bleeding, which is a known risk factor for endometriosis

Progestins

Progestins may exert an antiendometriotic effect by causing initial decidualization of endometrial tissue followed by atrophy. They can be considered a good second choice for the treatment of endometriosis because they are as effective in reducing ASRM scores and pain as OCs and have a lower cost and a lower incidence of side effects than that of danazol or GnRH analogs.

Medroxyprogesterone acetate (MPA) has been the most studied agent and is effective in relieving pain starting at a dose of 30 mg/day and increasing the dose on the basis of clinical response and bleeding patterns.

Alternatively, norethindrone at a dose of 5 mg/day is similarly effective.

Side effects of progestins include nausea, weight gain, fluid retention, and breakthrough bleeding due to hypoestrogenemia. Depression and other mood disorders are a significant problem in ~1% of women taking these medications.

Local progesterone treatment of endometriosis-associated dysmenorrhea with a levonorgestrel-releasing intrauterine system (IUS; Mirena)

over 12 months resulted in a significant reduction in dysmenorrhea, pelvic pain, and dyspareunia; a high degree of patient satisfaction; and a significant reduction in volume of rectovaginal endometriotic nodules.

In the future, progesterone antagonists and progesterone receptor modulators may suppress endometriosis on the basis of their antiproliferative effects on the endometrium, without risk of hypoestrogenism or bone loss as after GnRH treatment.

Gonadotropin-releasing hormone agonists

GnRH agonists bind to pituitary GnRH receptors and stimulate LH and FSH synthesis and release. However, the agonists have a much longer biological half-life (3–8 hours) than that of endogenous GnRH (3.5 minutes), resulting in the continuous exposure of GnRH receptors to GnRH agonist activity. This causes a loss of pituitary receptors and downregulation of GnRH activity, resulting in low FSH and LH levels.

Consequently, ovarian steroid production is suppressed, providing a medically induced and reversible state of pseudomenopause. This results in atrophy of the ectopic endometrial tissue.

The side effects of GnRH agonists are a result of the hypoestrogenism caused and include hot flashes, vaginal dryness, reduced libido, and osteoporosis (6–8% loss in trabecular bone density after 6 months of therapy). To prevent these, "add-back therapy in the form of HRT can be used. A GnRH agonist should always be used in the add-back therapy in the treatment of endometriosis.

Danazol

Pharmacological properties of danazol include suppression of GnRH, direct inhibition of steroidogenesis, increased metabolic clearance of estradiol and progesterone, direct antagonistic and agonistic interaction with endometrial androgen and progesterone receptors, and immunological attenuation of potentially adverse reproductive effects.

The multiple effects of danazol produce a high-androgen, low-estrogen environment that does not support the growth of endometriosis, and the amenorrhea that is produced prevents new seeding of implants from the uterus into the peritoneal cavity. The significant adverse side effects of danazol are related to its androgenic and hypoestrogenic properties.

The most common side effects include weight gain, fluid retention, acne, oily skin, hirsutism, hot flashes, atrophic vaginitis, reduced breast size, reduced libido, fatigue, nausea, muscle cramps, and emotional instability. Deepening of the voice is another potential side effect that is non-reversible.

Danazol is not more effective than other available medications to treat endometriosis and is therefore not commonly used.

Aromatase inhibitors

Treatment of rats with induced endometriosis using the nonsteroidal aromatase inhibitor fadrozole hydrochloride or YM511 resulted in dose-dependent volume reduction of the endometriosis transplants, but these products have not been used in published human studies.

Table 16.2 Side-effect profile of drugs used to treat endometriosis

Drug treatment	Side effects
NSAIDs, e.g., mefenamic acid	Gastric irritation
Combined oral contraceptives	Nausea, migraines, increased risk of thromboembolism
Progestogens, e.g., norethisterone	Fluid retention, bloating, and breast tenderness
Synthetic androgens, e.g., danazol	Androgenic, e.g., acne, weight gain
Gonadotropin-releasing hormone agonists	Menopausal symptoms, osteoporosis (these can be countered with use of "add-back" therapy with HRT)

Endomteriosis expresses the aromaste gene, enabling it to make its own endogenous estrogen and fuel its own growth. Endometriosis resistant to GnRH treatment may produce its own local estrogen.

Aromatase inhibitors (letrozole 5 mg/day) have been shown to be very effective in the treatment of endometriosis.

Aromatase inhibitors also result in increased pituitary FSH production due to the reduced estrogen feedback. Aromatase inhibitors must be used concurrently with agents that suppress hypothalamic–pituitary function such as GnRH analogs, OCs and progesterone. They are therefore most useful as second-line additions to the drug treatment (see Table 16.2 for side-effect profiles).

Further reading and information

ACOG practice bulletin. (2000). Medical management of endometriosis. Number 11, December 1999 (replaces Technical Bulletin Number 184, September 1993). Clinical management guidelines for obstetrician-gynecologists. *Int J Gynaecol Obstet* 71:183.

Endometriosis society: http://www.eshre.com/emc.asp

ESHRE guidelines for the diagnosis and treatment of endometriosis: http://guidelines.endometriosis.org/

Kennedy S, Bergqvist A, Chapron C, et al. (2005). ESHRE guideline for the diagnosis and treatment of endometriosis. *Hum Reprod* 20:2698.

McVeigh E, Koninckx PR (2005). Surgery for advanced endometriosis. In: Bonnar J, ed. *Recent Advances in Obstetrics and Gynaecology 23*. London: Royal Society of Medicine Press.

Mol BW, Bayram N, Lijmer JG, Wiegerinck MA, Bongers MY, Van der Veen F, Bossuyt PM (1998). The performance of CA-125 measurement in the detection of endometriosis: a meta-analysis. *Fertil Steril* 70(6):1101–1108.

Chapter 17

Intrauterine insemination

Introduction *152*
Methods *152*
Principle *152*
Indications *153*
IUI for mild male factor infertility *153*
IUI for unexplained infertility *153*
Cost-effectiveness *154*
Conclusions *154*
Further reading *154*

Introduction

Intrauterine insemination (IUI) involves the timed introduction of selected sperm into the uterine cavity. This is performed around the time of ovulation in unstimulated or stimulated cycles.

The usual indications for IUI are mild male-factor fertility problems or idiopathic (unexplained) infertility.

Methods

Three main methods are in use for the preparation of a fresh semen sample for IUI:
- Density gradient centrifugation
- Swim-up
- Washing in combination with centrifugation

Of these, density gradient centrifugation is reported to be the most efficient.

Following sperm preparation, the sample is introduced in the peri-ovulatory period into the uterine cavity using a standard catheter designed for this purpose. One insemination per treatment cycle has been shown to be as effective as two inseminations per cycle given 24 hours apart.

Principle

IUI was originally suggested for the treatment of mild male-factor infertility. The purpose of the laboratory treatment of the semen sample is to provide an "improved" sample by selecting actively motile sperm in an increased density. This sample can then be safely inserted into the uterine cavity through the cervix, thus placing a bolus of concentrated motile sperm closer to the available egg(s).

Indications

Mild male-factor (sperm count <20 but >5 million/mL and/or progressive motility <50% but >20%) infertility and idiopathic (unexplained) infertility are the two main indications for IUI.

The criteria for using IUI for the treatment of mild male-factor infertility vary from clinic to clinic, but generally IUI is used if the semen is of sufficient quality for there to be 1–5 million motile sperm available after sperm preparation. Less than 1 million motile sperm should indicate the use of in vitro fertilization (IVF) and intracytoplasmic sperm injection (ICSI) rather than IUI.

IUI is widely used for the empirical treatment of idiopathic infertility in both stimulated and unstimulated cycles. The combination of IUI with stimulated cycles, although improving pregnancy rates, is often accompanied by unacceptable multiple pregnancy rates. This suggests that the additional efficacy of stimulating the ovaries before IUI for unexplained infertility is due to multifollicular development, although correction of an undetected subtle defect in ovulatory function is also a possible contributory factor.

Male factor infertility is also effectively treated with assisted reproductive technologies (ART). ART can be offered as primary therapy in all couples with significant male-factor infertility.

IUI for mild male-factor infertility

IUI is more successful than both timed intercourse and intracervical insemination in couples with mild male infertility, whether in stimulated or natural cycles.

A systematic review of the literature revealed no significant difference between the results of IUI in stimulated and unstimulated cycles (pregnancy rates 13.7% vs. 8.4% per cycle, respectively) for this indication.

IUI for unexplained infertility

IUI with gonadotropin stimulation for this indication has proved to be more effective than gonadotropins alone.

Stimulated cycles in combination with IUI are more effective than unstimulated cycles in terms of pregnancy rates but are often accompanied by unacceptable multiple-pregnancy rates.

IUI + hMG (pregnancy rate 18% per cycle) was found to be more effective than IUI + CC (6.7%) and IUI in a natural cycle (4%) in an analysis of 45 reports. However, there was a resultant increase in multiple gestation.

Cost-effectiveness

For unexplained infertility, gonadotropin-stimulated cycles for IUI produce the best pregnancy rates but the highest multiple-pregnancy rates.

When compared with IUI in unstimulated cycles, the price of medication and the possible need for neonatal treatment of prematurely delivered multiple pregnancies raise the question of cost-effectiveness. The higher cost of medication and higher cost of multiple gestation make gonadotropin/IVF less cost-effective than milder stimulation while also providing higher success rates and more rapid concentration.

Recent studies suggest that IVF/ET (ET, embryo transfer) may be even more cost-effective because of its higher success rate and the ability to more precisely control the rate of multiple gestation.

Conclusions

IUI is a reasonably effective treatment for mild male-factor and idiopathic infertility.

It is generally reported that ovarian stimulation with gonadotropins improves results for unexplained infertility when combined with IUI for this indication. This combination is superior to use of gonadotropins alone or IUI alone.

For the treatment of mild male-factor infertility, gonadotropin stimulation before IUI does not significantly improve results.

The problem of unacceptable multiple-pregnancy rates using gonadotropin stimulation with IUI may be overcome by using a mild stimulation protocol and strict criteria for withholding hCG or by the use of IVF/ET.

Further reading

Cohlen BJ, Vanderkerckhove P, te Velde ER, Habbema ID (2000). Timed intercourse versus intrauterine insemination with or without ovarian hyperstimulation for subfertility in men. *Cochrane Database Syst Rev* 2000(2):CD000360.

Goverde AJ, McDonnell J, Vermeiden JP, Schats R, Rutten F, Schoemaker J (2000). Intrauterine insemination or in-vitro fertilization in idiopathic sub-fertility and male subfertility: a randomised trial and cost-effectiveness analysis. *Lancet* 355:13–18.

Chapter 18

In vitro fertilization and associated assisted conception techniques

Introduction *156*
Factors affecting the outcome of IVF *157*
Number of embryos transferred *158*
Procedures used during IVF *159*
Intracytoplasmic sperm injection *163*
Oocyte donation *163*
Complications of IVF *164*
Preimplantation genetic diagnosis (PGD)/preimplantation genetic screening (PGS) *165*
Follow-up of children born as a result of assisted reproduction *166*
Further reading and information *166*

Introduction

In vitro fertilization (IVF) refers to the extracorporeal fertilization of an oocyte. The term is, however, more loosely used to refer to the whole process of ovarian stimulation, oocyte retrieval, IVF, and embryo transfer (ET).

IVF-ET was initially developed to treat women with tubal infertility; now it is an established treatment for a wide variety of infertility diagnoses, including unexplained infertility. A number of factors should be considered for patient selection:

- Is there adequate ovarian reserve? Indications for this are age of the female and her early follicular (day 2–4) FSH level. As female age increases (>36 years) and as FSH rises (>10 IU/L), ovarian response to exogenous FSH stimulation will decrease.
- Are there any underlying medical, surgical, or psychological problems, e.g., severe renal disease or bowel adhesions secondary to Crohn's disease such that oocyte retrieval is not possible or safe?
- Is pregnancy safe for the woman and fetus? Are there any concerns over the welfare of the mother or child?

Factors affecting the outcome of IVF

The single most important prognostic factor for successful IVF is the female age, as shown in Fig. 18.1.

Before IVF is commenced, a female over the age of 35 should have her FSH level measured in the early follicular phase. This will give some indication as to the ovarian reserve anddegree of success of treatment.

The consumption of more than one unit of alcohol per day reduces the effectiveness of assisted reproduction procedures, including IVF treatment. It has also been shown that maternal and paternal smoking can have a similar adverse effect on success rates.

An elevated body mass index (BMI) >30 will not only decrease the chance of IVF working but also increase the miscarriage rate of a subsequent pregnancy.

Recent studies have demonstrated that the presence of hydrosalpinges may decrease the implantation rate of embryos following IVF. RCTs have shown that the removal of these hydrosalpinges prior to IVF increases the success rate.

The effect of stress on fertility and IVF has been and continues to be under study. To date, the evidence suggests that stress does not affect the outcome of IVF.

The psychological welfare of the IVF couple, however, should be cared for along with their physiological welfare. Counseling services should be available before, during, and after this stressful intervention.

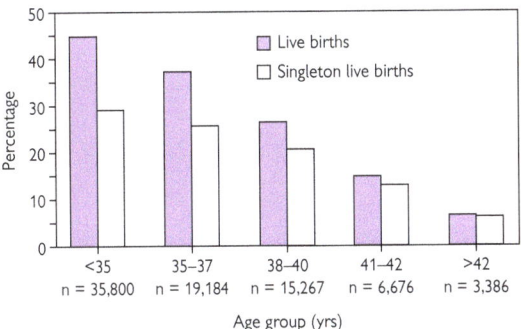

Fig. 18.1 Percentage of transfers resulting in live births and singleton live-births for assisted reproductive technology procedures performed among women who used freshly fertilized embryos from their own eggs, by patients' age group in 2006. The highest percentage of live births was about 45% among women under 35 years old. The lowest was approximately 7% for those more than 42 years old.
Source: Centers for Disease Control and Prevention. Sunderam S, Chang J, Flowers L, et al. (2009). Assisted reproductive technology surveillance—United States, 2006. *MMWRMorb Mortal Wkly Rep*58(SS05):1–25.

Number of embryos transferred

The widespread use of assisted reproductive technologies has caused an exponential increase in the multiple-pregnancy rates. In the United States, the incidence of triplet and higher-order pregnancies quadrupled from 1337 births in 1980 to 6737 births in 1997.

These pregnancies are at significant risk of perinatal and maternal morbidity and mortality, with considerable medical, social, and financial implications. Neonatal deaths are 7 times greater for twins and 23 times greater for triplets and higher-order pregnancies than for singleton pregnancies. The stillbirth rate is 3 times greater for twins and >4 times greater for triplet and higher-order pregnancies than that forsingletons.

Mothers are at increased risk of pre-eclampsia, anemia, ante- and post-partum hemorrhage and preterm labor, while fetuses are at increased risk of congenital malformation, intrauterine growth restriction, and complications of prematurity.

Cerebral palsy is 5 times more common in twins and 17 times more common in triplets.

The desire to increase the pregnancy rate through the transfer of increasing numbers of embryos must be balanced against this background. In the United States, the Society for Assisted Reproductive Technology (SART) and American Society for Reproductive Medicine (ASRM) guidelines recommendthat up to two embryos be transferred in women under the age of 40 years old and three embryos in women over the age of 40 years.

In a couple with good prognosis, elective single embryo transfer should be considered.

Procedures used during IVF

The IVF treatment cycle can be broken down into several different parts:
- Ovarian stimulation
- Ooctye retrieval
- In vitro fertilization
- Embryo transfer
- Luteal support

Ovarian stimulation

To obtain a number of oocytes, exogenous stimulation of the ovaries is required. If this is done without control of the hypothalamic–pituitary–ovarian axis, premature luteinization and ovulation may occur.

Attempts have been made to carry out "natural" IVF cycles with no ovarian stimulation or pituitary modulation. This method, however, leads to high cancellation rates due to a premature LH rise, as well as few embryos, with an ongoing pregnancy rate <10% per cycle. There is also no control over the timing of oocyte retrieval; this needs to be performed 26–28 hours after detection of the endogenous LH surge. Therefore, this method is still relatively expensive, as it requires monitoring, oocyte retrieval, and laboratory work.

The basis of modern IVF is the transvaginal retrieval of mature oocytes from gonadotropin-stimulated ovaries on the background of pituitary suppression.

Problems with premature LH rise led to the use of GnRH agonists and, more recently, GnRH antagonists. Initially, GnRH agonists were started with ovarian stimulation ("flare" or short protocol), but more commonly they are used for 2–3 weeks alone to achieve pituitary suppression (long protocol) followed by exogenous gonadotropins for ovarian stimulation.

Types of agonist

Endogenous GnRH contains 10 peptides with a half-life of a few minutes. Exogenous GnRH agonists have an increased half-life of several hours because of increased lipophilicity.

The continuous administration of GnRH agonists (daily or depot application) initially causes LH and FSH hypersecretion (flare), which is followed after a period of ~10 days by desensitization of the pituitary and profound suppression of LH and FSH. This results in the inhibition of ovarian steroidogenesis and follicular growth.

The agonist may be used in a number of different protocols.

Short (flare)
- Agonist started on cycle day 1
- Flare of pituitary output of gonadotropins
- Exogenous gonadotropins started on day 2
- Agonist continued until day of hCG

This protocol is sometimes used for women with reduced ovarian reserve. There is, however, no good evidence that this is better than other protocols, and it may actually be worse.

Microdose
- The theory is that reduced pituitary suppression will allow increased follicular response.
- Contraceptive pill pretreatment is needed.
- A low dose of daily agonist is started.

Long protocol
- This is the most established and widely used protocol.
- GnRH agonist suppresses pituitary production and release of gonadotropins.
- Initially there is flare of gonadotropin release until suppression occurs.
- GnRH agonists can be given by depot injection or daily SC or nasally. They are started in either the mid-luteal or early follicular phase.
- Pituitary suppression generally is achieved after 10–21 days. It is confirmed by the presence of withdrawal bleed, low serum estradiol level (<150 pmol/L), and/or ultrasound evidence of thin endometrium (<5 mm). If not suppressed, then look for an ovarian cyst that will need to be aspirated (this may occur as the result of the initial flare).

Alternatively, high-dose progestogens can be administered, which work by further suppressing pituitary gonadotropin release. Despite prolonged administration of GnRH agonist ± cyst aspirations, some women fail to achieve pituitary suppression. Options include canceling the cycle and restarting with antagonists.

Mid-luteal vs. early follicular agonist start
- Pregnancy rates are the same.
- There is a chance of starting the agonist during a natural conception cycle with mid-luteal start. This has not been shown to be detrimental to the pregnancy.
- There is ahigher rate of cyst formation with early follicular start.
- Cysts form in response to the initial flare effect of the agonist. Inactive (no raised estrogen level) cysts are not detrimental to outcome. If estrogen level is raised, the cysts should be aspirated transvaginally under ultrasound guidance.

Antagonists

Unlike GnRH agonists, the antagonists do not induce an initial hypersecretion of gonadotropins, but instead cause an immediate and rapid reversible suppression of gonadotropin secretion. The principal mechanism of action of GnRH antagonists is competitive occupancy of the GnRH receptor. The administration of a third-generation antagonist(e.g., cetrorelix and ganirelix) will result in the suppression of LH (~70%) and FSH (~30%)serum levels after ~6 hours.

The main benefits of antagonists over agonists are as follows:
- There is no need for prolonged administration as with a GnRH agonist since pituitary suppression is achieved within hours of administration.
- Protocols are either flexible or fixed start and single or multiple dose. With flexible start, the antagonist is started when the leading follicle is 14 mm in diameter. With fixed start, the antagonist is started on day 7 of stimulation without using ultrasound monitoring (thus regardless

of follicular size). While pregnancy rates are similar between the two approaches, the total gonadotropin dose is higher with a fixed start.

Comparison of protocols (Cochrane reviews)
Depot GnRH agonist vs. daily GnRH agonist
The use of a depot GnRH agonist compared with that of a daily agonist results in deeper pituitary suppression and an increased total dose of gonadotropins, with a longer duration of stimulation but no difference in clinical pregnancy rates.

The use of GnRH antagonists compared with that of agonists also results in a lower rate of severe ovarian hyperstimulation syndrome (OHSS), a lower rate of coasting/cycle cancellation, and a lower total dose and duration of gonadotropin stimulation.

Short-agonist vs. long-agonist protocols
In unselected patients (i.e., not poor responders), the use of short (flare), protocols results in a significantly lower pregnancy rate.

Urinary-derived and recombinant gonadotropins
Gonadotropin preparations in use are either urinary derived or recombinant. The recombinant preparations are either pure FSH (follitropin-α or β) or pure LH. Urinary products contain different amounts of LH activity depending on the particular preparation.

There does not appear to be any difference between urinary or recombinant gonadotropins in terms of live-birth rate per cycle.

LH activity
Some LH activity is required for optimal folliculogenesis (two-cell two-gonadotropin model).

Only 1% of follicular LH receptors need to be occupied for full LH effect. Therefore, the circulating levels of LH required are low.

LH does not need to be added to stimulation protocols using recombinant FSH in women with an intact pituitary, as pituitarysuppression is not absolute.

The degree of pituitary suppression is greater when depot GnRH agonist is used. Under these circumstances, some exogenous LH may be beneficial.

Exogenous LH is needed for hypopituitary women (two-cell two-gonadotropin model).

FSH dose selection
The main factors to consider with FSH dose selection are as follows:
- Ovarian reserve. The lower the ovarian reserve, the higher the gonadotropin dose.
- BMI. Overweight women require a higher dose.
- Previous ovarian response to stimulation, including poor response and OHSS
- Polycystic ovaries. The presence of ovaries with polycystic morphology, regardless of whether other aspects of PCOS, such as anovulation or hirsutism, are present, is a risk factor for OHSS, and so the FSH dose should be reduced. A starting dose of 150IU is prudent for the first cycle.

For women with normal ovarian reserve and without polycystic ovaries, starting doses of 150–250 IU result in similar numbers of oocytes retrieved and similar pregnancy rates.

Monitoring

Monitoring of follicular response can be assessed with serumestradiol levels (which represents follicular granulosa cell activity) and the number and diameters of follicles measured with transvaginal ultrasound.

The use of estradiol measurements in addition to scan monitoring does not improve the rate of pregnancy or reduce OHSS rates.

hCG is given when at least three follicles of ≥17–18mm diameter are present. The hCG mimics the mid-cycle LH surge. Recombinant LH is also available, although no advantages have been demonstrated.

Oocyte collection

In the early days of IVF, the oocyte collection was done laparoscopically and required general anesthesia.

Today, oocyte aspiration is usually performed transvaginally under ultrasound guidance with IV sedation and analgesia, unless the ovary is not assessable by this route or if gamete intrafallopian tube transfer (GIFT) is taking place.

Embryo transfer and embryo freezing

This occurs usually on day 3 post–oocyte insemination or post-ICSI. It may be delayed until blastocyst formation on day 5 in the attempt to select better morphological embryos and thus improve the pregnancy rate per embryo transfer.

The procedure involves passing a fine catheter through the cervix. This may be done under ultrasound guidance, as this appears to increase the pregnancy rate. Replacement of embryos into a uterine cavity with an endometrium of <5mm thickness is unlikely to result in a pregnancy and is therefore not recommended.

Surplus embryos may be frozen and subsequently used in a frozen embryo transfer replacement cycle (FERC). In general, the better the morphological quality of the embryo at freezing, the better the survival rate from the freeze–thaw process.

Pregnancy rates following FERCs tend to be slightly lower than those with the equivalent fresh embryo transfer cycle.

Luteal phase support

As a result of the downregulation of the hypothalamic–pituitary axis, there will be insufficient endogenous LH to stimulate ovarian progestone production following oocyte collection. Progesterone in the form of vaginal suppository or IM injection is required for the weeks following oocyte collection and embryo transfer to ensure receptivity of the endometrium.

The routine use of hCG (as an LH replacement) for luteal support is not recommended because of the increased likelihood of OHSS.

Intracytoplasmic sperm injection

This procedure was first carried out in 1993. Since that time, ICSI has been performed extensively. The recognized indications for treatment by ICSI include
- Obstructive azoospermia
- Nonobstructiveazoospermia

In addition, treatment by ICSI should be considered for couples in whom a previous IVF treatment cycle has resulted in failed or very poor fertilization. Before considering treatment by ICSI, couples should undergo appropriate investigations, both to establish a diagnosis and to enable informed discussion about the implications of treatment.

When the indication for ICSI is a severe deficit of semen quality or nonobstructive azoospermia, the man's karyotype should be established. When a specific genetic defect associated with male infertility is known or suspected (e.g., cystic fibrosis), couples should be offered appropriate genetic counseling and testing.

Testing for Y chromosome microdeletions should not be regarded as a routine investigation before ICSI. However, it is likely that a significant proportion of male infertility results from abnormalities of genes on the Y chromosome involved in the regulation of spermatogenesis, and couples should be informed of this.

Oocyte donation

The use of donor oocytes may be considered in managing fertility problems associated with the following conditions:
- Premature ovarian failure
- Gonadaldysgenesis, including Turner's syndrome
- Bilateral oophorectomy
- Ovarian failure following chemotherapy or radiotherapy
- Certain cases of IVF treatment failure where there is a severely diminished ovarian reserve

Oocyte donation should also be considered in certain cases where there is a high risk of transmitting a genetic disorder to the offspring. Before donation is undertaken, oocyte donors should be screened for both infectious and genetic diseases.

Oocyte donors should be offered information regarding the potential risks of ovarian stimulation and oocyte collection. Oocyte recipients and donors should be offered counseling regarding the physical and psychological implications of treatment for themselves and their genetic children, including any potential children resulting from donated oocytes.

"Egg-sharing" is a program whereby women undergoing IVF offer to share half of the oocytes retrieved at collection with another women who requires egg donation. Both couples entering into this arrangement should be counseled about its particular implications.

Complications of IVF

The short-term risks of IVF include the following:
- OHSS
- Trauma
- Infection
- Stress

The most common problem is OHSS. Other less common complications are pelvic infection (0.4%), intraperitoneal bleeding (0.2%), and adnexaltorsions (0.13%). Trauma accounts for ~0.1–0.2% and may involve problems such as puncture of an ovarian cyst, trauma to bowel, trauma to pelvic vessels, and even trauma to the ureter.

Ovarian hyperstimulation syndrome (OHSS)

This is the best recognized complication of ovarian stimulation for IVF or ovulation induction. It remains incompletely understood, but the luteinizing trigger is undoubtedly an essential feature in the problem.

If the luteinizing trigger is withheld, the excessive ovarian response should regress without OHSS resulting. The worst cases tend to be associated with pregnancy, since if there is no pregnancy, the hCG stimulus soon regresses. Moderate OHSS occurs in ~3–4% of cycles and risk of severe OHSS is ?0.1–0.2%.

With the massive ovarian enlargement that occurs after luteinization in this syndrome, the clinical picture becomes complex. The problems include hypoproteinemia, tension ascites, pleural effusion, hemoconcentration, oliguria and electrolyte imbalance, a hypercoagulable state, liver dysfunction, and, in some cases, death.

Once the syndrome has developed, early admission is appropriate, although there are limited measures that can be employed. These include gentle IV hydration, anticoagulation with heparin, metabolic support with protein replacement to maintain the circulating volume, paracentesis to relieve the ascites, and, in some very serious cases, termination of pregnancy.

Preimplantationgenetic diagnosis (PGD)/ preimplantationgenetic screening (PGS)

The ability to culture embryos to the blastocyst stage (day 5) mean that there is time for genetic testing. The blastomeres are totipotent on day 3, and biopsy of the embryo, removing one cell, may be performed without harming the developmental potential of the embryo. This cell may be tested using polymerase chain reaction (PCR) to identify a known genetic defect previously identified in a prospective parent. Only unaffected embryos are subsequently transferred on day 5.

Preimplantation genetic screening is similarly used to identify chromosome abnormalities in embryos, typically using fluorescence in situ hybridization (FISH). This technique has been shown to reduce pregnancy rates in prospective study, due to elimination of mosaic embryos and false-positive results.

Newer technology, such as a day 5 biopsy with comparative genomic hybridization (CGH), may offer better results. However, this is not typically available.

Follow-up of children born as a result of assisted reproduction

The course of pregnancies and the health of children born as a result of assisted conception technologies are two of the most important outcome parameters of the quality of the techniques. There is ongoing discussion as to whether these outcomes are poorer with assisted reproduction than with spontaneous conception.

It was initially thought that this difference was predominantly the result of a higher incidence of multiple pregnancies in this group or was the result of increased maternal age. A recent study on subfecundity and neonatal outcome in the Danish national birth register also concluded that subfecundity in itself may be associated with an increased risk of neonatal death.

Shortly after the introduction of ICSI in the mid-1990s, it was noted that children born following ICSI had a slightly increased incidence of abnormalities. On closer examination, in the vast majority of these cases there was already an existing genetic or chromosomal predisposition toward an abnormality on the paternal side.

It has been reported that genomic imprinting (an epigenetic phenomenon by which the expression of a gene is determined by its parental origin and only one allele of the imprinted gene is expressed) may be disrupted during IVF. It has been reported that Beckwith–Wiedemann syndrome (an imprinting disorder) has a 6-fold increase in incidence against a background incidence of ~1.3 per 100,000 newborns.

Whatever the factors are, it does appear that IVF pregnancies are at an increased risk of perinatal mortality and related perinatal outcomes (prematurity and low gestation weight). Whether these factors are related to aspects of the treatment, closer follow-up of the child, the underlying features that the couples bring to the pregnancy, or a mixture of all three, is not yet clear.

Further reading and information

National Institute for Health and Clinical Excellence (NICE) report into fertility investigation and treatment: www.nice.org.uk/pdf/CG011niceguideline.pdf

Part 2

Contraception and Family Planning

19	Fertility and fertility awareness	**169**
20	Male contraception	**181**
21	Vaginal methods	**187**
22	The combined oral contraceptive (COC)	**193**
23	Progestogen-only pill (POP)	**223**
24	Injectables	**231**
25	Contraceptive implants	**239**
26	Intrauterine contraception	**247**
27	Postcoital contraception	**261**
28	Sterilization	**269**
29	Special considerations	**275**

Chapter 19

Fertility and fertility awareness

Introduction *170*
Sex and relationships education (SRE) *170*
Sexually transmitted Diseases *171*
Features of the ideal contraceptive *172*
Relative effectiveness of the available methods *173*
Eligibility criteria for contraceptives *175*
Fertility awareness and methods for the natural regulation of fertility *176*

Introduction

We now shift to a consideration of "the other side of the coin": fertility control rather than its enhancement. Most women who seek contraception are healthy and young and present fewer problems than those over age 35, teenagers, and those with intercurrent disease.

The combined oral contraceptive (COC) is too often seen as synonymous with contraception. There are many new or improved reversible alternatives to the COC and the condom.

Some women, after years of using contraception, have difficulty conceiving. Not unreasonably, they may blame the contraceptive. Fortunately, it is rare that the methods per se are truly causative (beyond allowing the woman to get older before she tries to get pregnant). Even the injectable depot medproxyprogesterone acetate (DMPA) is fully reversible, although in some women it may considerably delay return of ovulation.

Indeed, it is the *lack of* contraception, leading to septic abortion, that causes much (tubal) infertility in some parts of the world—not to mention non-use of the condom, causing pelvic inflammatory disease (PID).

Sex and relationships education (SRE)

Whether being taught about or seeking advice on sex, relationships, contraception, pregnancy, and parenthood, young people are entitled to
- Accessible information
- Confidential counseling
- Nonjudgmental approach
- Unbiased support and guidance that recognizes the diversity of their cultural and faith traditions.

Their own views should be listened to, the educator respecting the opinions and choices of young people being counseled. Choices include abstinence and safer sex. Discussion of sexual safety should include both contraception and risks of sexually transmitted diseases (STDs).

A significant proportion of early postpubertal menstrual cycles are not fertile. Hence adolescents who have unprotected sex shortly after puberty commonly "get away with it," leading to a false sense of security later on, when their fertility is much higher.

Typically, their pill-taking is very haphazard. Teenagers should thus be offered one of the long-acting reversible contraceptives (LARCs) far more frequently than is currently the case in most settings, even if their first thought has been to ask for "the pill."

Injectables and implants are usually preferable to copper intrauterine devices (IUDs) because they are more readily initiated (i.e., no vaginal procedure) and may provide some protection against pelvic infection—although IUDs are only relatively contraindicated.

The levonorgestrel intrauterine system (LNG-IUS) may also be appropriate.

Yet for many young women, the most acceptable initial method of contraception currently remains a modern, low-estrogen OC.

With all these methods, there should be appropriate counseling and condom use to avoid STDs.

Sexually transmitted diseases

The prevalence in the United States of gonorrhea, chlamydia, and syphilis is rising.

The most common conditions now are human papillioma virus (HPV) and chlamydia (>10% of sexually active teenagers have acquired *Chlamydia trachomatis*), but almost all sexually transmitted diseases (STDs) are becoming more common.

In the United States, women at higher risk of infection (particularly with *C. trachomatis*) are those
- Aged under 25
- With a partner change in the previous 12 weeks
- With more than one partner in the past 12 months

Sexual history should be seen as part of the initial consultation for *all* contraceptives, not just the intrauterine ones, and include the following questions:
- "When did you last have sex?" followed at once by
- "When did you last have sex with someone different?"

The sexually active of all ages should be advised about minimizing their risk of STDs, including the human immunodeficiency virus (HIV). *It is essential to promote the condom as an addition to the selected contraceptive whenever infection risk exists.*

Contact tracing

Where an STD has been identified, contact screening is best done through a genitourinary medicine (GUM) clinic. In some states, there is mandatory protocol when certain STD testing is positive.

Features of the ideal contraceptive

Consideration of the factors affecting successful use of contraception by young people lends support to the need for as many of the 10 features listed in Box 19.1 as possible.

Box 19.1 The ideal contraceptive

- 100% effective (with the default state as contraception)
- 100% convenient (forgettable, noncoitally related)
- 100% safe, free of adverse side effects (neither risk nor nuisance)
- 100% reversible, ideally by self
- 100% maintenance-free, meaning needing absolutely no medical or provider intervention (with potential pain or discomfort)—whether initially or during usage or to achieve reversal
- 100% protective against STDs
- Having other noncontraceptive benefits, especially to the dis-"eases" of the menstrual cycle
- Cheap, easy to distribute
- Acceptable to every culture, religion, and political view
- Used by or at least clearly visible to the woman, who most needs to know it has worked!

It is difficult to decide the best priority order for these factors, although the first six bullets are clearly paramount.

Relative effectiveness of the available methods

Failure rates of contraceptive methods are usually expressed as failures per 100 woman-years (Pearl Index). A figure of 10 per 100 woman-years for a "perfect user" (see below) means the following:
- In a population of 100 users, 10 women might be expected to conceive in the first year of use.
- Or one woman would have an "evens" chance of having an unplanned pregnancy after 10 years of its use.

In Table 19.1, "perfect use" means the method is used both consistently and correctly, whereas "typical use" means what it says—note the huge difference in percentage conceiving after 1 year between the two types of use for the combined pill (0.3 vs. 8).

Fig. 19.1 shows current usage of the present mix of methods.

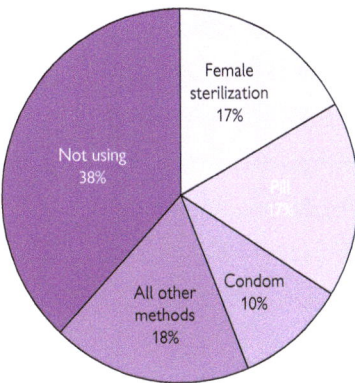

Figure 19.1 Percent distribution of women aged 15-44 years, by current contraceptive status: United States, 2006-2008.
Source: Mosher WD, Jones J. Use of contraception in the United States: 1982-2008. National Center for Health Statistics. Vital Health Stat 23(29). 2010.

Table 19.1 Percentage of women experiencing an unintended pregnancy during the first year of use of contraceptive

Method	Typical use	Perfect use
No method	85	85
Spermicides	29	18
Withdrawal	27	4
Periodic abstinence	25	
Calendar		9
Ovulation method		3
Symptothermal[1]		2
Postovulation		1
Cap + spermicide		
Parous women	32	26
Nulliparous women	16	9
Sponge		
Parous women	32	20
Nulliparous women	16	9
Diaphragm	16	6
Condom		
Female	21	5
Male	15	2
Combined pill and minipill	8	0.3
Combined hormonal patch	8	0.3
Combined hormonal ring	8	0.3
DMPA	3	0.3
Combined injectable	3	0.05
IUD		
ParaGard® (banded copper T)	0.8	0.6
Mirena® (LNG-IUS)	0.1	0.1
LNG implants	0.05	0.05
Female sterilization	0.5	0.5
Male sterilization	0.15	0.1

Emergency contraceptive pills: treatment initiated within 72 hours after unprotected intercourse reduces the risk of pregnancy by at least 75%.

Lactational amenorrhea method: LAM is a highly effective, *temporary* method of contraception.

Note: This table in WHOMEC, 3rd edition, 2004, has been adapted from the source document by changing the title, changing the trade names of methods to generic names, and by modifying footnotes.
[1] This refers to the cervical mucus method supplemented by calendar calculation in the preovulatory and basal body temperature charting in the postovulatory phases. See pp. 176 and 177.
Source: Trussell J (2004). Contraceptive efficacy. In: Hatcher RA, Trussell J, Stewart F, Nelson A, Cates W, Guest F, Kowal D. *Contraceptive Technology: Eighteenth Revised Edition.* New York: Ardent Media.

Eligibility criteria for contraceptives

The World Health Organization (WHO) system for classifying contraindications

The WHO system for classifying contraindications to contraceptive use is described in the WHO documents *Medical Eligibility Criteria for Contraceptive Use* (WHOMEC) (3rd ed., 2004, ISBN: 9241562668) and *Selected Practice Recommendations for Contraceptive Use* (WHOSPR) (ISBN: 9241545666). See http://www.who.int/reproductive-health.

Box 19.2 WHO classification of contraindications to use of contraceptives *

WHO 1. A condition for which there is no restriction for the use of the contraceptive method
  A is for Always usable

WHO 2. A condition where the advantages of the method generally outweigh the theoretical or proven risks
  B is for Broadly usable

WHO 3. A condition in which the theoretical or proven risks usually outweigh the advantages, so an alternative method is usually preferred. Yet, respecting the patient or client's autonomy, if she accepts the risks and rejects or should not use relevant alternatives, given the risks of pregnancy, the method can be used with caution or sometimes with additional monitoring
  C is for Caution/Counseling, if used at all

WHO 4. A condition that represents an unacceptable health risk
  D is for DO NOT USE at all

Clinical judgment is required, always in consultation with the contraceptive user, especially (1) in all WHO 3 conditions, or (2) if more than one condition applies. As a working rule, two WHO 2 conditions move the situation to WHO 3; and if any WHO 3 condition applies, the addition of either a 2 or a 3 condition normally means WHO 4, i.e., do not use.

*Modified by the author.

Fertility awareness and methods for the natural regulation of fertility

These are capable of being much more reliable than the old calendar rhythm (see the excellent Web site, http://www.fertilityuk.org, and associated review by Pyper and Knight[1]) if there is correct and consistent use. However, these methods still remain very unforgiving of imperfect use.

Short notes on the background physiology
- An average fertile man's ejaculate contains ~300–400 million sperm.
- The acidic vaginal environment can kill sperm in a matter of hours; however, in estrogen-primed cervical mucus and upper genital tract fluid, average sperm survival is ~3 days.
- In rare individuals or rare cycles in which favorable mucus appears early, fertilization can be as long as 7 days after ejaculation.
- The average fertilizable lifespan of the egg(s) after ovulation is ~17 hours, with a range up to a maximum of 24 hours.
- Adding the lifetime of the sperm to that of the egg gives a "fertile window" of 7–8 days, whose length is rather constant. But its time of onset shows intra- and interindividual variation.
- Maximum reliability will require many days of abstinence, especially early in the cycle. For maximum efficacy with any of the methods, unprotected intercourse should preferably, following good evidence of ovulation, be confined to the days after the ovum can no longer be fertilized.

Markers of ovulation
One marker is a rise in basal temperature that has been sustained for 72 hours at least 0.2°C above the preceding 6 days' values.

Another is that the mucus at the vulva becomes increasingly fluid, glossy, transparent, slippery, and stretchy, like raw egg white, under the influence of follicular estrogen. The peak mucus day can be recognized retrospectively as the last day with such features before the abrupt change to a thick and tacky type (under the influence of progesterone).

The postovulatory infertile phase is defined as beginning on the evening of the fourth day after the peak mucus day, provided this is also after the third day of the higher morning temperature readings.

Relying on *both* the above signals for the onset of the postovulatory infertile phase and using that alone for unprotected intercourse can give very acceptable failure rates of 1–3 per 100 woman-years.

The preovulatory infertile phase is much more difficult to identify with accuracy. The indicators are as follows:
- The first sign of any mucus at all, detected by either sensation or appearance

---

1 Pyper CM, Knight J (2001). Fertility awareness methods of family planning: the physiological background, methodology and effectiveness of fertility awareness methods. *J Fam Plann Reprod Health Care* 27:103–110.

- Calendar calculation of the shortest cycle minus 20 (or better yet, 21) to give the last "infertile" day, where at least six cycle lengths are known. This can be enhanced by the Doering rule, in which 7 days are subtracted from the earliest cycle day of documented temperature shift. Whichever of these two indicators comes first indicates the requirement to abstain.

Relying on both phases is only recommended to those who can accept a pregnancy, since calculations and mucus observations do NOT reliably predict ovulation.

The postpartum period and in the climacteric years
Temperature and mucus estimations are unreliable and/or give numerous false alarms, since some cycles are anovulatory, yet still there is sufficient estrogen to produce copious mucus.

Advantages of methods based on fertility awareness
- They are completely free from any known physical side effects for the user.
- They are acceptable to many with various religious and cultural views.
- The methods are under the couple's personal control (abstinence is always available!).
- The methods readily lend themselves to the additional use of an artificial method such as a barrier at the potentially fertile times, including during the less safe first "infertile" phase.
- Once established as efficient users, after proper teaching, no further expensive follow-up of the couple is necessary.
- Understanding of the methods can also help couples who then wish to conceive.

Problems and disadvantages
- In practice, *typical use* gives very high failure rates (25 per 100 woman-years according to Trussell, Table 19.1). This is almost entirely due to not following the Doering rule or calendar calculation.
- Conflicts and frustrations are reported, though interestingly enough, the majority of *established* users believe the method to be helpful to their marriage and relationship, rather than stressing it.
- A potential hazard is fetal abnormalities due to conceptions tending to result from fertilization involving aging gametes. The consensus after a number of studies is that this risk, if real, is negligible.

The lactational amenorrhea method (LAM)
Ovulation is delayed among women who fully or nearly fully breastfeed their babies. It usually takes between 1 and 3 months for a woman to begin to ovulate and for her cycle to return to normal after stopping breastfeeding.

LAM is an algorithm, as shown in Fig. 19.2, allowing a woman to determine whether she is comfortable relying on her pattern of infant feeding and menstruation to predict anovulation or whether she should add an additional method of contraception.

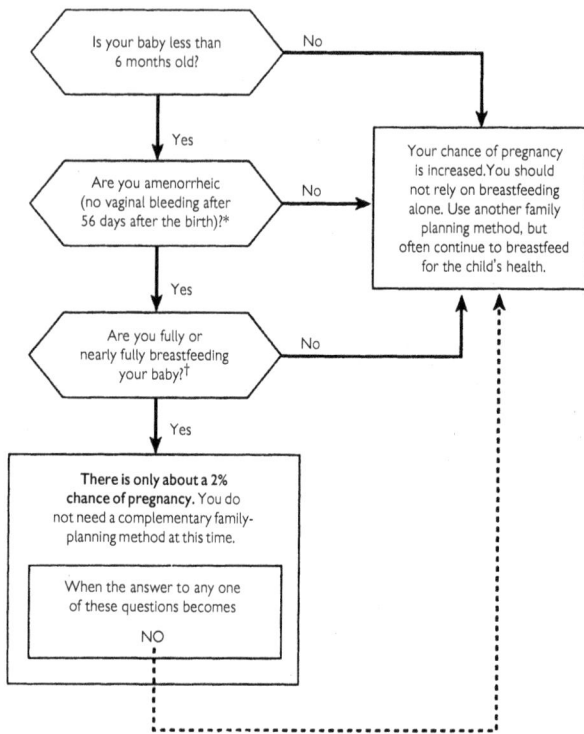

Figure 19.2 Algorithm for the lactational amenorrhea method (LAM). *Spotting that occurs during the first 56 days is not considered to be menstruation. "Nearly" full breastfeeding means that the baby obtains 100% of its nutrition from the mother alone, and certainly no solid food.
Reproduced from *The Pill*, part of the Facts series. 6th edition. By permission of Oxford University Press.

Additional methods for postpartum use

The OC should be avoided early in lactation, as it may inhibit lactation and alter the quality of the milk. Otherwise, the COC is a suitable choice postpartum.

The progestone-only pill (POP) is preferable. This does not interfere significantly with lactation, and although traces may enter the milk, the quantity has been calculated (see Chapter 23) as equivalent to a baby getting just one pill over 2 years.

Spermicides or contraceptive sponges, though not generally effective enough for recommendation to young people, are strong enough as adjunctive methods while the LAM rules are valid.

Condoms (including the female condom) are useful for first intercourse postpartum and until other methods are established. Caps and diaphragms may be refitted at 5–6 weeks, and this is always necessary after a full-term pregnancy, even after Caesarean section.

The injectable DMPA, aside from slightly higher milk levels (which seem to be harmless to the infant), may be a preferable progestogen-only method for women who might be short-term breastfeeders and unreliable POP takers but want high efficacy right through weaning and thereafter. It does no detectable harm to the quality of breast milk and may even improve the quantity.

Implanon® or implantable contraceptives are another option.

The IUD or IUS is easily inserted at 4–6 weeks postpartum or 6–8 weeks after a Caesarean section, but the uterus is still soft and great care is necessary. Earlier insertion is more likely to lead to expulsion.

Sterilization procedures performed in the postpartum period carry an extraoperative failure rate and emotional risks (including greater risk of regret). Surgery for either partner is usually, and preferably, delayed for a few months.

Chapter 20

Male contraception

Coitus interruptus *182*
Male condoms *183*
The male pill *184*
Vasectomy *185*

Coitus interruptus

This is the earliest form of reversible birth control (mentioned in Genesis and positively in Islamic texts); it is well described by its most common euphemism, "withdrawal" (before ejaculation, ensuring that all sperm are deposited outside the vagina).

Effectiveness of coitus interruptus

Its pregnancy rate is reported as 8 per 100 woman-years of exposure. Trussell gives a 4% failure rate in the first year of "perfect use" (see Table 19.1).

Sperm are found at low density in some men in the pre-ejaculate. A more probable cause of failure is either the partial ejaculation of a larger quantity of semen occurring a short while before the final male orgasm or withdrawal during male orgasm rather than before it starts.

It can therefore be useful to advise couples who want to continue using the method that they might use a spermicide as well (never instead).

Advantages
- Free, requires no prescription
- Always available
- No side effects

Disadvantages
- Intercourse is incomplete, and either or both partners may find the method decidedly unsatisfying.

Conclusion

Coitus interruptus is almost never proposed as a contraception to a couple. If they volunteer that this is already their usual method, other options should always be discussed.

If all alternatives are unacceptable, the additional use of spermicide (e.g., as a pessary or sponge) should be suggested.

Male condoms

Condoms are the only proven barrier to the transmission of HIV. Condoms are second in usage to the OC under the age of 30 and to sterilization above that age.

Effectiveness

With "perfect use" the failure rate is 2%, and typical use leads to 15% of couples conceiving in the first year.

The main reason for failure is either intermittent non-use or incorrect use: mainly through the escape of a small amount of semen either before or after the condom is in place for the main ejaculation, rather than rupture.

Advantages and indications

Aside from acceptable, potentially good efficacy, advantages of male condoms include the following:
- Useful protection against all sexually transmitted diseases (STDs), including HIV and human papilloma virus (HPV)
- Easy to obtain, even at odd hours
- No need to see a health care provider
- No medical risks and no supervision required
- Visual proof of having "worked"
- Helps delay premature ejaculation for some men
- Good for infrequent intercourse

Problems and disadvantages

- To many people, condoms seem intrusive; alteration of sensations in the penetrative phase of sex are reported by the male, sometimes by both partners.
- There is poor efficacy in typical use, largely from lack of care or consistency. This is often related to the first problem mentioned above. Hence, It is often best combined with a medical and more effective method.
- Condoms need to be readily available. Planning is needed.
- They can slip off or rupture in use.
- Rubber (not plastic) condoms may be seriously weakened by oil-based chemicals. All users need warning of this risk. Water-based and silicone lubricants are OK.

Lubricants with the spermicide nonoxinol 9 should be avoided with any condom, since there is now evidence showing that it can increase HIV transmission (see p. 190). Moreover, it provides no detectable increase in condom efficacy.

The male pill

The male pill is still very much a work in progress and has yet to be marketed. The main problems are as follows:
- Male contraception is biologically more difficult to achieve than female contraception. There is no single regular event like ovulation that can be stopped.
- A male pill must not affect libido, must give extremely good protection against pregnancy, and must be as free as possible from side effects.
- There is a special risk here that interference with the production of the sperm might be incomplete. So if one sperm were damaged by whatever the treatment might be, yet managed to fertilize an egg, this might result in a birth defect.
- Spermatogenesis takes ~70 days. Thus any male pill operating on this manufacturing process will take at least 2 months to become effective. It also means that there must be a long recovery period after stopping the method.

Research has focused either on
- Stopping the production of sperm or
- Inactivating or blocking them once produced.

The former approach is the closest to producing a viable, marketed method, by combining a progestogen via injection or implant with an androgen, a long-acting analog of testosterone. This blocks both FSH and LH, the LH therefore switching off production of testosterone. But the androgen content is titrated to a level to preserve libido and drive without the drive turning into aggression.

Vasectomy

For more discussion of male and female sterilization, see Chapter 28.

Bilateral vasectomy is a safe and effective method of male sterilization. In the United States it is underutilized despite being less invasive than tubal ligation.

Because the sperm itself makes up a very small proportion of an ejaculation, vasectomy does not significantly affect the volume, appearance, and texture of the ejaculate. Two negative semen analyses (2–4 weeks apart and >12 weeks since the procedure) are the norm after the surgical procedure to ensure effectiveness.

In counseling, several steps are necessary before valid consent can be obtained. See Chapter 28 for further discussion. The process should at least include the following:
- An assessment of the patient's contraceptive needs and discussion of alternative methods
- A general discussion of the surgical technique, tailored to the individual
- A frank and honest discussion of the risks and specific complications associated with vasectomy
- As with any medical intervention, only patients of sound mind and capable of understanding these issues are able to give valid consent.

Early failure rates of vasectomy are generally <1% (see Table 20.1), but the effectiveness of the operation and rates of complications vary with the level of experience of the surgeon performing the operation and the surgical technique used. Although late failure (caused by recanalization of the vasa deferentia) is very rare, it has been documented.

Table 20.1 Failure rates (first year)

Perfect use	<0.1%
Typical use	0.15%
Usage	
Duration effect	Permanent
Reversibility	Often, but not always
User reminders	Additional methods required until two negative semen samples
Clinic review	None

Chapter 21

Vaginal methods

Female condoms *188*
Caps and diaphragms *189*
Spermicide (nonoxinol) *190*

Female condoms

The female condom comprises a polyurethane sac with an outer rim at the introitus and a loose inner ring, whose retaining action is similar to that of the rim of the diaphragm. It thus forms a well-lubricated (with silicone) secondary vagina.

- *Effectiveness:* failure rate is 5% among "perfect" users after 1 year.
- *Duration of use:* used near or at the time of intercourse, whereas the diaphragm or cap must be left in place for at least 6 hours after intercourse. Appropriate for both short-term and long-term use. Reuse of the female condom is not recommended. Women can use barrier contraceptives throughout their reproductive years.
- *Parity limitations:* there are no restrictions on use for nulliparous or parous women, although parous women may experience higher rates of pregnancy with the diaphragm and cap.

Advantages
- Useful protection against all sexually transmitted diseases (STDs), including HIV and HPV
- Available over the counter, along with a well-illustrated leaflet
- Completely resistant to damage by any chemicals with which it might come into contact
- Usable if either party is allergic to rubber
- The penetrative phase of intercourse can feel more normal to a man than when a male condom is used.
- Uniquely among condoms, it can be put in place before the man has an erection.

Disadvantages
Couples should be forewarned of
- The definite possibility that the penis may become wrongly positioned between the condom and the vaginal wall.

Caps and diaphragms

These create a vaginal barrier to sperm either in the upper vagina (diaphragms) or at the cervix itself.
- Effectiveness: failure rate is 5 per 100 "perfect" users, rising to 16 per 100 typical users after 1 year.

Spermicide is recommended for use as well, because no mechanical barrier is complete. Possible toxic effects of nonoxinol to the vaginal wall have become a real concern (see below).

Advantages
- Once initiated, many couples express surprise at the simplicity of these vaginal barriers. They are best reserved for couples in a stable relationship where sexual activity takes on a relatively regular pattern and conception would not be seen as a disaster.
- All may be inserted well ahead of coitus and so used without spoiling spontaneity.
- There is very little reduction in sexual sensitivity, as the clitoris and introitus are not affected and cervical pressure is still possible.

Disadvantages
- Rather moderate efficacy, plus lack of complete protection against the viral STDs such as HIV
- Concerns about spermicide safety (see next section)
- Perceptions that they are a hassle to learn to use

Fitting and follow-up

One-to-one training is crucial, both in the process of fitting the diaphragm and cervical caps and in teaching a woman how to use it correctly, backed up by an appropriate leaflet.

The fitting of diaphragms should be checked initially after 1–2 weeks of trial and rechecked routinely postpartum or whenever there is more than 3 kg gain or loss in weight.

If either partner returns complaining that they can feel a diaphragm during coitus, the fitting must be urgently checked. It could be too large or too small, the retropubic ledge may be insufficient to prevent the front from slipping down the anterior vagina, or, most seriously with respect to efficacy, the item may wind up being regularly placed in the anterior fornix.

Recurrent cystitis may be linked to pressure from a diaphragm's anterior rim and hence often improves with a vault or cervical cap, which does not apply pressure on the anterior vagina.

Spermicide (nonoxinol)

Although invaluable as an adjunct to caps and diaphragms and for some couples using coitus interruptus long term, spermicide used alone—whether as creams, jellies, pessaries or foams—is simply not acceptably reliable. However, good effectiveness has been reported in women whose fertility is already reduced.

Contraceptive sponges share the advantage with spermicides of being sexually very convenient and unobtrusive in use, but once again lack sufficient efficacy (see Table 19.1) for most young, fertile women. Yet all of these methods can be good for defined populations (see Box 21.1)

Box 21.1 Spermicide use for defined populations

The Today™ sponge or other spermicidal products may be good choices in the following cases:
- For women >50 years of age if still experiencing bleeds after stopping the COC (see p. 278) and for 1 year after menopause (i.e., the duration for which contraception is still advised), regardless of whether they use HRT
- For women aged >45 if they have oligoamenorrhea
- During lactation, as an alternative to the POP
- During continuing secondary amenorrhea, unless a COC is being used anyway to treat hypoestrogenism
- As an adjunct to other contraception, e.g., spermicides may be useful as a supplement for couples who choose to continue using coitus interruptus or withdrawal as their main method
- For those who are nearly but not quite ready for a first or subsequent child

Disadvantages

- The currently available spermicide nonoxinol is certainly absorbed from the vagina, but there is no proof that there is no systemic harm, congenital malformations, or spontaneous abortions as a result.
- Occasionally, sensitivity to spermicides arises.
- More seriously, when used by Nairobi sex workers four times a day for 14 days, nonoxinol released from pessaries caused erythema and colposcopic evidence of minor damage to the vaginal skin. Subsequent clinical trials have confirmed an increased risk of HIV transmission with use of spermicidal products using nonoxinol.[1] High risk of HIV infection is therefore WHO 4 (see p. 175) for this substance, whether used alone or with a vaginal barrier.

---

[1] Wilkinson D, Tholandi M, Ramjee G, Rutherford GW (2002). Nonoxynol-9 spermicide for prevention of vaginally acquired HIV and other sexually transmitted infections: systematic review and meta-analysis of randomised controlled trials including more than 5000 women. *Lancet Infect Dis* 2:613–617.

However, the vagina is believed to be able to recover between applications when nonoxinol is used in the manner and at the kind of average coital frequency of appropriately counseled diaphragm or cap users. So it remains good practice to recommend nonoxinol-9 for normal contraceptive use, whether alone or with diaphragms or cervical caps, but not with condoms (📖 p. 183).

Chapter 22

The combined oral contraceptive (COC)

Mechanism of action *194*
Benefits versus risks *195*
Tumor risk and COCs *196*
Cardiovascular disease *199*
WHO Eligibility criteria for COCs *205*
The pill-free interval (PFI) *211*
Drug interactions *212*
Other relevant drugs *213*
Counseling and ongoing supervision *216*
Stopping COCs *220*
Other combined methods *221*
Pill follow-up *221*
Congenital abnormalities and fertility issues *222*

Mechanism of action

The mechanism of action of a COC is as follows:
- Primarily prevents ovulation
- Secondary contraceptive effects on the cervical mucus and impeding of implantation

This makes the method highly effective in "perfect" use (see Table 19.1), but it removes the normal menstrual cycle and replaces it with a cycle that is user produced and based only on the end. This cycle has minimal medical significance, can be deliberately postponed or made infrequent, and, if it fails to occur, once pregnancy is excluded, poses no problem.

The pill-free time is the contraception-deficient time, which has great relevance to advice for the maintenance of the COC's efficacy.

Benefits versus risks

Contraceptive benefits of COCs
- Effectiveness
- Convenience, not intercourse related, "forgettability"
- Reversibility

Noncontraceptive benefits of COCs
At times such benefits may be the principal indication for use of this method (e.g., in the treatment of dysmenorrhea in a not yet sexually active teenager).
- Reduction of most menstrual cycle disorders: less heavy bleeding, thus less anemia, and less dysmenorrhea; regular bleeding, the timing of which can be controlled (no COC taker need have periods on the weekends; upon request, she may tri-cycle and thus bleed only a few times a year): fewer symptoms of premenstrual tension overall; no ovulation pain
- Reduced risk of cancers of the ovary and endometrium (see next section) and very probably also of colorectal cancer
- Fewer functional ovarian cysts because abnormal ovulation is prevented
- Fewer extrauterine pregnancies because normal ovulation is inhibited
- Reduction in pelvic inflammatory disease (PID)
- Reduction in benign breast disease
- Fewer symptomatic fibroids
- Probable reduction in thyroid disease, whether over- or underactive
- Probable reduction in risk of rheumatoid arthritis
- Fewer sebaceous disorders (with estrogen-dominant COCs)
- Possibly fewer duodenal ulcers (not well established)
- Reduction in *Trichomonas vaginalis* infections
- Possible lower incidence of toxic shock syndrome
- Continuous use beneficial in long-term suppression of endometriosis
- No toxicity in overdose
- Some obvious beneficial social effects, to balance suggested negatives

Risks of COCs
- Tumors: breast, cervical, liver
- Venous thromboembolism (VTE)
- Arterial diseases: acute myocardial infarction (AMI), hemorrhagic stroke (HS), and ischemic stroke (IS)

Tumor risk and COCs

Breast cancer
COC users can be reassured of the following:
- An odds ratio of 1.24 signifies an increase of 24% only while women are taking the COC, diminishing to zero after discontinuation, over the next few years.
- Beyond 10 years after stopping, there is no detectable increase in breast cancer risk for former COC users.
- The cancers diagnosed in women who use or have ever used COCs are clinically less advanced than in those who have never used COCs and are less likely to have spread beyond the breast.
- These risks are not associated with duration of use, the dose, or the type of hormone in the COC, and there is no synergism with other risk factors for breast cancer (e.g., family history). See Table 22.1.
- If 1000 women use the pill until age 35, by age 45 this model shows that there will be, in all, 11 cases of breast cancer. Importantly, however, only one of these cases is extra (pill-related); the others would have arisen in a control group of never-users.

Clinical implications
Women with benign breast disease (BBD) or with a family history of a first-degree relative with breast cancer under age 40 have a larger background risk than all women, but only the same as women slightly older than their current age who are free of the risk factor (no restriction to use).

If the woman with BBD had a breast biopsy, the histology should be obtained: if epithelial atypia (premalignant) was found, caution should be exercised.

If a woman develops carcinoma of the breast, COCs should be discontinued, and women with a history of this cancer should usually avoid COCs.

Cervical cancer
The COC acts as a cofactor for the human papilloma virus (HPV) types 16 and 18, the principal carcinogen in cervical cancer, speeding transition

Table 22.1 Increased risk of developing breast cancer while taking the pill and in the 10 years after stopping

User status	Increased risk
Current user	24%
1–4 years after stopping	16%
5–9 years after stopping	7%
10 years + an ex-user	No significant excess

Reprinted from Hertzen HV, Piaggio G, Peregoudov A, et al. (2002). Low dose mifepristone and two regimens of levonorgestrel for emergency contraception: a WHO multicentre randomised trial. *Lancet* 360:1803–1810, with permission from Elsevier.

through the stages of cervical intraepithelial neoplasia (CIN). In this respect, it is similar to but certainly weaker than cigarette smoking.

Clinical implications
Prescribers must ensure that COC users are adequately screened according to accepted guidelines.

It is acceptable practice to continue COC use during the careful monitoring of any abnormality or after definitive treatment of CIN.

Liver tumors

There is an increased relative risk of benign adenoma or hamartoma. However, the background incidence is so small (1–3 per 1 million women per year) that the COC-attributable risk is minimal.

Three case–control studies also support the view that the rare primary hepatocellular carcinoma is minimally less rare in COC users than in controls.

Choriocarcinoma or all gestational trophoblastic disease

Clinical implications
Women are advised not to conceive
- For 6 months after hCG levels are normal, and
- For at least 12 months from conclusion of any chemotherapy (there is risk of recurrent disease and teratogenic effects of the chemotherapy).

So what contraception should be used?
- Fortunately, while hCG levels are >5000 IU/L, ovulation is very improbable, so barrier methods should be effective. These are the first choice for what is usually a short time.
- The progestogen-only methods are acceptable while hCG is elevated, and emergency contraception (EC) is also permitted.
- Combined hormonal methods can be used as soon as hCG concentrations are normal.
- Intrauterine methods are not recommended until a normal menstrual cycle is established.

Carcinomas of the ovary and of the endometrium

Both occur definitely less frequently in COC users.

A protective effect can be detected in ex-users for up to 15 years and for carcinoma of the ovary if use lasts over 30 years. In both cases the risk is about halved among women who use COCs for 15 years.

Suppression in COC users of ovulation and of normal mitotic activity in the endometrium are the accepted explanations for these findings.

Clinical implications
It would be reasonable for a woman known to be predisposed to either of these cancers to use the COC primarily for this protective effect.

Colorectal cancer

There are very suggestive data from a number of studies that the pill also *protects* against this cancer.

Women who are apparently cured by local surgery for neoplasia of the ovary and cervix and for malignant melanoma may all use COCs.

The bottom line when counseling COC takers is as follows: Populations using the pill may develop different benign or malignant neoplasms from control populations, but it does not appear from computer modeling studies that the overall risk of neoplasia is increased. See Fig. 22.1.

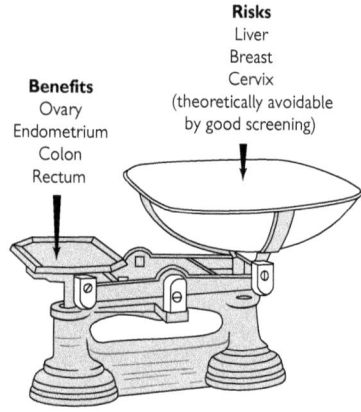

Figure 22.1 Cancer and the pill: a balance. Based on a figure from *The Pill*, part of the Facts series. 6th edition. By permission of Oxford University Press.

Cardiovascular disease

Venous thromboembolism (VTE)
The spontaneous incidence of VTE in healthy nonpregnant women (not taking any oral contraceptive) is about 5 cases per 100,000 women per year. The incidence in users of second-generation pills is about 15 per 100,000 women per year of use. The incidence in users of third-generation pills is about 25 cases per 100,000 women per year of use: this excess incidence has not been satisfactorily explained by bias or confounding.

The level of all of these risks of VTE increases with age and is likely to be increased in women with other known risk factors for VTE such as obesity.

Arterial diseases: acute myocardial infarction, hemorrhagic stroke, and ischemic stroke

Acute myocardial infarction (AMI)
If current or past pill-takers are nonsmokers, studies find a nil or extremely small added risk of AMI.

Hemorrhagic stroke (HS), including subarachnoid hemorrhage
There is no increased risk due to use of the COC under age 35 unless there is also a risk factor such as hypertension (odds ratio [OR] 10) or smoking (OR 3). The risk increases with age, and this effect is magnified by current COC use, but with no effect of past use or long-duration use.

Ischemic stroke (IS)
Here there is a detectable increase in the OR due to pill taking in the range of 1.5 to a maximum of 2. Much of this risk seems to be focused within the subpopulation that suffers from migraine with aura (see p. 208). The OR for hypertension is 3, and for smoking, also 3.

Effect of dose and type of hormone
It is believed, though has never been proven, that the modern low-estrogen pills help minimize the arterial risks. Whether the type of progestogen in the COC separately affects (as it can only do in those with risk factors) the arterial conditions listed above is still uncertain.

Prescribing guidelines
Prescribers should always take a comprehensive personal and family history and check the woman's body mass index (BMI) and blood pressure (BP) to exclude absolute and relative contraindications to the use of COCs (see pp. 205-207).

A personal history of definite VTE remains an absolute contraindication to any hormonal method containing ethinylestradiol (EE), combined with any progestogen.

The risk factors for risk of future VTE and arterial wall disease must be assessed (see Tables 22.2 and 22.3):
- Smoking is an independent risk factor for VTE, as is arterial disease.
- Alone, one risk factor from either Table 22.2 or Table 22.3 is a relative contraindication, unless it is particularly severe.

CHAPTER 22 **The combined oral contraceptive (COC)**

Table 22.2 Risk factors for venous thromboembolism (VTE) and contraindications for COC use

Risk factor	Absolute contraindication WHO 4	Relative contraindication WHO 3	WHO 2	Remarks
Personal or family history (FH) of thrombophilias, or of venous thrombosis in sibling or parent	Past VTE event; or identified clotting abnormality in this person, whether hereditary or acquired FH of a defined thrombophilia or *idiopathic* thrombotic event in parent or sibling <45 and thrombophilia screen not (yet) available	FH of thrombosis in parent or sibling <45 with recognized precipitating factor (e.g., major surgery postpartum) and thrombophilia screen not available	FH of thrombotic event in parent or sibling <45 with or without a recognized precipitating factor and *normal thrombophilia screen* in parent or sibling ≥45 or FH in second-degree relative (classified WHO 2 but tests not indicated)	*Idiopathic* VTE in a parent or sibling <45 is an indication for a thrombophilia screen if available. The decision to undertake screening in other situations (including where there was a recognized precipitating factor) will be unusual because this is very cost-ineffective—it might be done on clinical grounds, in discussion with the woman Even a normal thrombophilia screen cannot be entirely reassuring, as some predispositions are not yet known.
Overweight—high body mass index (BMI)	BMI ≥40	BMI 30–39	BMI 25–29	See Note 5
Immobility	Bed-bound, with or without major surgery; or leg fractured and immobilized	Wheelchair life, debilitating illness	Reduced mobility for other reason	Minor surgery, such as laparoscopic sterilization, is WHO 1

Varicose veins (VVs)	Current superficial vein thrombosis in the upper thigh Current sclerotherapy for VVs (or imminent VV surgery)	History of superficial vein thrombosis (SVT) in the lower limbs, no deep vein thrombosis	SVT does not result in pulmonary embolism, although this past history indicates using some caution (WHO 2) in case it might be a marker of future VTE risk. Uncomplicated
Cigarette smoking	≥15 cigarettes per day	< 15 cigarettes per day	On balance, the literature suggests a VTE risk from smoking, though less than the arterial disease risk it causes
Age >35	>51	35–51 if age is sole risk factor	

[1] A single risk factor in the relative contraindication columns indicates use of LNG/NET pill, if any COC is used.

[2] Beware of synergism: more than one factor in either of relative contraindication columns. As a working rule, two WHO 2 conditions make WHO 3; and if WHO3 applies (e.g., BMI 30–39), addition of either a WHO 3 or WHO 2 (e.g., reduced mobility) condition normally means WHO 4 (do not use).

[3] Acquired (nonhereditary) predispositions include positive results for anti-phospholipid antibodies—definitely WHO 4 since they also increase the risk of arterial events (Table 22.4)

[4] There are also important acute VTE risk factors, which need to be considered in individual cases:
- Dehydration from any cause
- Long-distance flights
- Major and all leg surgery.

CHAPTER 22 **The combined oral contraceptive (COC)**

Table 22.3 Risk factors for arterial disease and contraindications for COC use

Risk factor	Absolute contraindication	Relative contraindication		Remarks
		WHO 4	WHO 3	
Family history (FH) of atherogenic lipid disorder or of arterial CVS event in sibling or parent	Identified familial hyperlipidemia in this person, persisting despite treatment	FH of known familial lipid disorder or of *idiopathic* arterial event in parent or sibling <45 and client's lipid screening result: Not available or Confirmed and responding to treatment	Client has the less problematic common hyperlipidemia and is responding well to treatment FH of arterial event with risk factor (e.g. smoking) <45, and lipid screen not available	FH of premature (<45) arterial CVS disease without other risk factors, or a known atherogenic lipid disorder in a parent or sibling, is an indication for fasting lipid screen, if available (then check with laboratory about clinical implication of abnormal results) Despite any FH, normal lipid screen in client is reassuring and means WHO 1 (in contrast to thrombophilia screening)
Cigarette smoking	≥40 cigarettes per day	15–39 cigarettes per day	<15 cigarettes per day	Cutoffs here are somewhat arbitrary.
Diabetes mellitus (DM)	Severe, long-standing or DM complications (e.g., retinopathy, renal damage, arterial disease)	Not severe/labile and no complications, young patient with short duration of DM		DM is always at least WHO 3 for the COC (safer options are available)
Hypertension (consistently elevated BP, with properly taken measurements)	Systolic BP ≥160mmHg Diastolic BP ≥95mmHg	Systolic BP in range >140–159 mmHg Diastolic BP >90–95 mmHg On treatment for essential hypertension, with good control	BP regularly at upper limit of normal (i.e., near to 140/90 mmHg) Past history of pre-eclampsia (WHO 3 if also a smoker)	

Overweight, high BMI	BMI ≥ 40	BMI 30–39	BMI 25–29	High BMI increases arterial as well as VTE risk
Migraine	Migraine with aura Migraine without aura if attacks last >72 hr + no overuse of medication	Migraine without aura plus a strong added arterial risk factor	Migraine without aura	Relates to *thrombotic* stroke risk Triptan treatment does not affect the category
Age >35	>35 if a continuing smoker Age >51 for all others, even if risk factor-free	35–51, if ex-smoker	Age 35–51 if free of all risk factors (yet even safer options are available)	In all persistent smokers, age >35 is best classified as WHO 4 Ex-smokers are WHO 3 because arterial wall damage may persist; but UKMEC permits WHO 2 after 1 year of not smoking

[1] Beware of synergism: more than one factor in either of relative contraindication columns. As a working rule, two WHO 2 conditions make WHO 3; and if WHO 3 applies, (e.g., smoking >15 cigarettes/day), addition of either a WHO 3 or WHO 2 (e.g., age 35) condition normally means WHO 4 (as in Table 22.3).

[2] The pill seems to have a negligible, though not nil, adverse effect in arterial disease, unless there is a risk factor.

[3] WHO numbers also relate to use for contraception: use of COCs for medical indications such as PCOS often entails a different risk–benefit analysis, i.e., the extra therapeutic benefits might outweigh expected extra risks.

Hereditary predispositions to VTE (thrombophilias)
Almost the only indication for screening is a strong family history of one or more siblings or parents having had a spontaneous VTE under the age of 45. This justifies testing for the genetic predispositions, including factor V Leiden (the genetic cause of activated protein C resistance).

The woman's strong family history cannot be discounted, since all the predisposing abnormalities of the complex hemostatic system have yet been characterized.

Acquired predispositions to VTE (thrombophilias)
Antiphospholipid antibodies that increase both VTE and arterial disease risk (Table 22.3, Note 3) may appear in a number of connective tissue disorders, most commonly in systemic lupus erythematosus (SLE). If identified, they absolutely contraindicate COC use.

WHO eligibility criteria for COCs

Absolute contraindications to COCs or other combined methods (e.g., Evra)

1. Past or present circulatory disease
- Any past proven arterial or venous thrombosis
- Ischemic heart disease or angina or coronary arteritis (Kawasaki disease—this is WHO 3 after recovery)
- Severe or combined risk factors for venous or arterial disease (see Tables 22.3 and 22.4) can be WHO 4—though usually graded lower (as below).
- Atherogenic lipid disorders (get advice from an expert, as indicated)
- Known prothrombotic states
- Abnormality of coagulation/fibrinolysis, i.e., congenital or acquired thrombophilias;
- From at least 2 (preferably 4) weeks before until 2 weeks after mobilization following elective major or leg surgery (do not demand that the COC be stopped for minor surgery such as laparoscopy); during leg immobilization (e.g., after fracture) or varicose vein treatment; and
- When going to high altitudes if there are added risk factors (otherwise WHO 3, see below)
- Migraine with aura (described on 📖 p. 208)
- Definite aura *without* a headache following
- Transient ischemic attacks
- Past cerebral hemorrhage
- Pulmonary hypertension, any cause
- Structural (uncorrected) heart disease such as valvular heart disease or shunts and septal defects are only WHO 4 if there is an added arterial or venous thromboembolic risk (persisting, if there has been surgery). Always discuss this with the cardiologist—this could be WHO 3, especially if the patient is always on warfarin. Important WHO 4 examples are as follows:
- Atrial fibrillation or flutter whether sustained or paroxysmal—or not current but high risk (e.g., mitral stenosis)
- Dilated left atrium (>4 cm)
- Cyanotic heart disease
- Any dilated cardiomyopathy, but not a past history of any type when in full remission (WHO 2)

In other structural heart conditions, if there is little or no direct or indirect risk of thromboembolism (this being the crucial point to check with the cardiologist), the COC is usable (WHO 3 or 2).

2. Disease of the liver
- Active liver cell disease (whenever liver function tests are currently abnormal, including infiltrations and cirrhosis)
- Past pill-related cholestatic jaundice (if in pregnancy can be WHO 3)
- Dubin–Johnson and Rotor syndromes (Gilbert's disease is WHO 2)

- Following viral hepatitis or other liver cell damage: but COCs may be resumed 3 months after liver function tests have become normal
- Liver adenoma, carcinoma
- Acute hepatic porphyrias; other porphyrias are usually WHO 3, but a nonsteroid hormone method is usually preferable.

3. History of serious condition affected by sex steroids or related to previous COC use
- SLE—also VTE risk
- COC-induced hypertension
- Pancreatitis due to hypertriglyceridemia
- Pemphigoid gestationis
- Chorea
- Stevens–Johnson syndrome (erythema multiforme), if COC associated
- Trophoblastic disease, but only until hCG levels are undetectable
- Hemolytic uremic syndrome (HUS) and thrombotic thrombocytopenic purpura (TTP). HUS in the past with complete recovery is generally WHO 2.

4. Pregnancy

5. Undiagnosed genital tract bleeding

6. Estrogen-dependent neoplasms
- Breast cancer
- Past breast biopsy showing premalignant epithelial atypia

7. Miscellaneous
- Allergy to any pill constituent
- Past benign intracranial hypertension
- Specific to Yasmin®

Because of the unique spironolactone-like effects of the contained progestogen drospirenone (DSP), this particular brand should be avoided, should any COCs be appropriate, in anyone at risk of high potassium levels (including severe renal insufficiency, hepatic dysfunction, and treatment with potassium-sparing diuretics).

8. Woman's anxiety about COC safety unrelieved by counseling

Several of the contraindications listed here (e.g., 4–5, 8) are not necessarily permanent contraindications. Moreover, in the past, many women were unnecessarily deprived of COCs for reasons now shown to have no link, such as thrush, or which would have positively benefited from the method, such as secondary amenorrhea with hypoestrogenism.

Relative contraindications to COCs

Unless otherwise stated, relative contraindications to COCs are WHO 2:
- Risk factors for arterial or venous disease (see Tables 22.3 and 22.4). These are WHO 2, sometimes WHO 3, provided that only one is present and not of such severity as to justify WHO 4.

- HUS (see above) in past history may be WHO 2 if there is complete recovery and is not pill associated (e.g., past *E. coli* 0157 infection as established cause of HUS)
- Diabetes (minimum category being WHO 3), hypertensive disease, and migraine all deserve separate discussion, below.
- Risk of altitude illness. This is not more probable because a climber is on COC, but if it occurs, in its most severe forms there may be venous or arterial thromboembolism or patchy pulmonary hypertension, either of which would contraindicate use of COCs. Hence, all women traveling to above 2500 m should be informed that the COC might increase the thrombotic component of severe arterial illness if that were to occur. For more details, see Barry and Pollard.[1]
- Sex steroid–dependent cancer in prolonged remission (WHO 3); prolonged is defined as after 5 years by WHO Medical Eligibility Criteria (MEC)
- Prime example is breast cancer
- Malignant melanoma any time post-diagnosis is WHO 2 for the pill.
- If a young (<40 years of age) first-degree relative has breast cancer (WHO 2)
- Established BBD
- During the monitoring of abnormal cervical smears (WHO 2)
- During and after definitive treatment for CIN (WHO 2)
- Oligo- or amenorrhea (COCs may be prescribed after investigation— may be WHO 1, use unrestricted, if the purpose is to supply estrogen in a woman needing contraception or to control the symptoms of PCOS)
- Hyperprolactinemia (WHO 3, but only for patients who are on specialist drug treatment and with close supervision)
- Most chronic congenital or acquired systemic diseases (see below) are WHO 2:
  - Sickle cell trait is WHO 1 but homozygous sickle cell disease is WHO 2 (although DMPA is preferred for this)
  - Inflammatory bowel disease is WHO 2, or WHO 3 if severe because of VTE risk in exacerbations
  - Otosclerosis (WHO 2)
  - Gallstones (WHO 3, but WHO 2 after cholecystectomy)
  - Very severe depression if there is a clear history of it being exacerbated by COCs (but unwanted pregnancies can be depressing!).
- Diseases that require long-term treatment with enzyme-inducing drugs are WHO 3 (COC usable, see below, but alternative contraception is preferred).

Alternatives to COCs in these cases would be POP or barrier methods.

Diabetes mellitus (DM)

Consider DM a WHO 3 condition even when there is no *known* diabetic tissue damage (cf. WHOMEC, which classes well-controlled DM as WHO 2).

---

1 Barry PW, Pollard AJ (2003). Altitude illness. *BMJ* 326:915–919.

Clinically, given the high arterial disease risk, progestogen-only pills (POPs) (often Cerazette®) or Implanon® are preferred alternatives.

Mercilon®, Femodette®, or Loestrin 20® (see above) are COC options, but for limited duration and under careful supervision. This would be for cases where there is no known arteriopathy, retinopathy, neuropathy, or renal damage, nor any added arterial risk factor such as obesity or smoking—all of which mean WHO 4—and preferably if the duration of the disease has been short (Table 22.4).

Hypertension

In most women on COCs, there is a slight increase in both systolic and diastolic blood pressure (BP) within the normotensive range: ~1% become clinically hypertensive, and the rate increases with age and duration of use. If BP is repeatedly >160/>95 mmHg, the method should be stopped. If it then normalizes, this pill-induced hypertension is WHO 4 for the future.

Past severe toxemia (pregnancy-induced hypertension) does not predispose to hypertension during COC use, but it is a risk factor for myocardial infarction (WHO 2), markedly so if the women also smokes (WHO 3).

Essential hypertension (not COC related), when well controlled on drugs, is WHO 3, i.e., the COC is usable but not preferred.

Migraine

Migraines can be defined by the answers to the following question: "During the last 3 months, did you have the following with your headaches?"

1. You felt *nauseated* or sick in your stomach.

2. You were *bothered by light* a lot more than when you don't have a headache.

3. Your headaches *limited your ability* to work, study, or do what you needed to do for at least 1 day.

Two "yes" answers means the diagnosis of migraine.

Migraine and stroke risk

Studies have shown an increased risk of ischemic stroke in migraine sufferers and in COC users; if combined, there is "summation" of risk.

There is good evidence of exacerbation of risk by arterial risk factors, including smoking and increasing age above 35 years.

The presence of aura before or even without the headache is the main marker of risk (WHO 4), not only for ischemic stroke but also for coronary artery disease and myocardial infarction. It seems increasingly likely that there is no significantly increased risk through having migraine without aura, though currently this is still classified as WHO 2.

Given that the 1-year prevalence of any migraine in women has been shown to be as high as 18%, it is crucial to identify the important subgroup with aura (1-year prevalence ~5%).

Migraine with aura

Taking this crucial history starts by establishing the timing: *neurological symptoms of aura begin before the headache itself* and typically last ~20–30 minutes, maximum 60 minutes, and stop before the headache does (which

may be very mild). Headache may start as aura is resolving or there may be a gap of up to 1 hour.
- Visual symptoms occur in 99% of true auras and hence should be asked about first.
- These are typically bright and affect part of the field of vision, on the same side in both eyes (homonymous hemianopia).
- Fortification spectra are often described, typically a bright scintillating zigzag line gradually enlarging from a bright center on one side, to form a convex C-shape surrounding the area of lost vision (which is a bright scotoma).
- Sensory symptoms are confirmatory of aura, occurring in around one-third of cases and rarely in the absence of visual aura—typically paresthesia spreading up one arm or one side of the face or the tongue. The leg is rarely affected. They are positive symptoms, *not loss of function*.
- Disturbance of speech may also occur, as nominal dysphasia.

Clinical implications—taking an aura history
- Ask the woman to describe a typical attack as it starts from the very beginning, including any symptoms before a headache. Listen to what she says but at the same time watch her carefully.
- A most useful sign that what she is describing is likely true aura is if she draws something like a zigzag line in the air with a finger to one or other side of her own head.

In summary, aura has three main features:
- Characteristic TIMING: onset BEFORE (headache) + duration ≤1 hour + Resolution before or with onset of headache
- Symptoms VISUAL (99%)
- Description VISIBLE (using a hand)

Absolute contraindications (WHO 4) to starting or continuing COC
- *Migraine with aura* or *aura without headache*. The *artificial estrogen* of the COC is what needs to be avoided (or stopped) to minimize the additional risk of a thrombotic stroke.
- Other migraines (even without aura) which are exceptionally severe in a COC taker and last >72 hours despite optimal medication
- All migraines treated with ergot derivatives, owing to their vasoconstrictor actions
- *Migraine without aura* plus multiple risk factors for arterial disease, or a relevant interacting disease (e.g., connective tissue diseases already linked with stroke risk)

In all the above circumstances, any of the *progestogen-only*, i.e., *estrogen-free*, hormonal methods may be offered immediately. Similar headaches may continue, but now without the potential added risk from prothrombotic effects of EE. Particularly useful choices are Cerazette®, Implanon®, the LNG-IUS, or a modern copper IUD.

Migraine: relative contraindications for the COC
WHO 2: the COC is "broadly usable" in the following cases:

- *Migraine without aura* and also without an important arterial risk factor from Table 22.3 and still under the age of 35. If these (or other "ordinary" headaches) occur only or mainly in the pill-free interval (PFI), tri-cycling the COC may help.
- *Use of a triptan drug* in the absence of important other contraindicating factors.
- *The occurrence of a woman's first ever attack of migraine without aura while on the COC.* A reasonable precaution is to stop the pill if she is seen during the attack. But after full evaluation of the symptoms, provided there were no features of aura or marked risk factors, the COC can be restarted later (WHO 2), with the usual counseling and caveats about future aura.

WHO 3: The COC is usable with caution and close supervision:
- Primarily is migraine without aura (common or simple migraine) with important risk factors for ischemic stroke present (i.e., when the patient is already WHO 3, migraine without aura adds little further risk).
- Secondly: a clear past history of typical migraine *with aura* >5 years earlier or only during pregnancy, with no recurrence, may be regarded as WHO 3. COCs may be given a trial, along with counseling and regular supervision and a specific warning that the onset of definite aura (carefully explained) means the user should
- Stop the pill immediately,
- Use alternative contraception, and
- Seek medical advice as soon as possible.

Differential diagnoses

It may be difficult to distinguish such relatively common, migraine associated transient ischemia from rare organic episodes—true transient ischemic attacks (TIAs) (e.g., due to paradoxical embolism, which is an established risk of an atrial septal defect or persistent foramen ovale). TIAs are more sudden in onset than migraine aura and last over an hour, without other migraine symptoms such as nausea.

A suspicion of TIA means the same as an actual one in practice, i.e., WHO 4—stop the pill immediately. But if an organic episode is a possibility, hospital investigation should also follow, including for the following features that are not typical of migraine:
- Focal epilepsy, severe acute vertigo, hemiparesis, ataxia, aphasia, unilateral tinnitus
- A severe unexplained drop attack or collapse
- Monocular blindness (black scotoma) could rarely be a retinal vascular event or a symptom of TIA—amaurosis fugax
- Progressive or persistent neurological symptoms (migraine is episodic with complete freedom from symptoms between attacks)

Why have pill-free intervals at all?

The pill-free week promotes a reassuring withdrawal bleed. If this is not seen as important, and to obtain certain other advantages, any woman may omit the PFIs and associated bleeds as a long-term option.

Seasonale is a dedicated packaging in the United States that provides four packets in a row, followed by a 7-day, pill-free week, such that the user has a bleed every 3 months (i.e., seasonally).

Lybrel (Wyeth Pharamceuticals) was recently approved as a continuous oral contraceptive containing no placebo. This may be particularly advantageous in woman with dysmenorrhea or endometriosis.

Clinical implications

In the short term, the gap between packets of monophasic brands is often omitted (upon request) to avoid a menstrual period on special occasions. Users of phasic pills who wish to postpone withdrawal bleeds must use the final phase of a spare packet or use pills from an equivalent formulation.

Breakthrough bleeding (BTB) may become a problem during longer active pill regimens. It may be that the COC for that woman is unable to maintain endometrial stability for so long.

One solution, provided a minimum of seven tablets have been taken since the last PFI (and it will usually be far more), is to advise at any time a definite 4- to 7-day break. Some women tolerate bi-cycling best, i.e., 42 days of continuous pill taking followed, depending on the indication, by a 4- to 7-day PFI.

Drug interactions

Drug interactions reduce the efficacy of COCs mainly by induction of liver enzymes, which leads to increased elimination of both estrogen and progestogen (Fig. 22.2). Additionally, in a very small (but unknown) minority of women, disturbance by certain broad-spectrum antibiotics of the gut flora that normally split estrogen metabolites that arrive in the bowel can reduce the reabsorption of reactivated estrogen.

According to WHOMEC, this effect is probably negligible clinically (but see below). It is certainly not a factor in the maintenance of progestogen levels and thus is irrelevant to the POP.

The most clinically important drugs with which interaction occurs are given in the lists below.

Enzyme inducer drugs (important examples) that interact with COCs

- Rifampicin, rifabutin
- Griseofulvin (antifungal)
- Barbiturates
- Phenytoin
- Carbamazepine
- Oxcarbazepine
- Primidone
- Topiramate (if daily dose >200mg)
- Modafinil
- Some antiretrovirals (e.g., ritonavir, nevirapine)—full details are obtainable from http://www.hiv-druginteractions.org
- St John's Wort (potency varies)

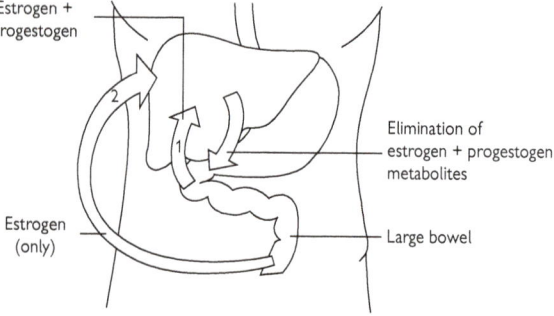

Figure 22.2 The enterohepatic recirculation of estrogen and its implications for drug interactions. (1) First absorption of both hormones, via the liver. (2) Reabsorption of some estrogen, but not progestogen. See text.

Other relevant drugs

None of the proton-pump inhibitors, including lansoprazole, is now regarded as having any clinically important enzyme induction effect.

Ethosuximide, valproate, and clonazepam, and most newer anti-epileptic drugs (including vigabatrin and lamotrigine), do not pose this problem.

Lamotrigine levels can be *lowered* by COCs, so starting a COC in a patient already taking this may result in poorer control of the epilepsy. Thus a small increment in the dose of lamotrigine is all that is required. There is no problem in giving lamotrigine to patients already taking a COC because the dose of lamotrigine is titrated as usual to the patient's needs.

Ciclosporin levels can be *raised* by COC hormones. The risk of toxic effects means blood levels should be measured in sex steroid users.

Drospirenone, the progestogen in Yasmin®, should not be used in women on potassium-sparing diuretics (risk of hyperkalemia).

Clinical implications

Short-term use of any interacting drug (enzyme inducer or antibiotic)
Recommended regimen:
- Additional contraceptive precautions are advised during the treatment and should then be continued for a further 7 days.
- If at the end of treatment there are fewer than seven tablets left in the pack (i.e., third week), the next PFI should be eliminated (skip any placebo pills).

Rifampicin is such a powerful enzyme inducer that even if it is given only for 2 days (e.g., to eliminate carriage of meningococci), increased COC elimination by the liver must be assumed for 4 weeks thereafter, i.e., as though it had been given long term (see below). The extra contraception (e.g. condoms) should be continued to cover all that time, plus the elimination of any expected PFIs.

Long-term use of antibiotics

The large-bowel flora responsible for recycling estrogens are reconstituted with resistant organisms within ~2 weeks. In practice, therefore, if COCs are commenced in a woman who has been taking a tetracycline long term, there is no need to advise extra contraceptive precautions.

There is a potential problem (now believed to involve very few women) in the reverse situation, i.e., when the tetracycline is first introduced to treat a long-term COC user. Even then:
- Extra precautions need only be sustained for a maximum of 21 days (which includes the usual 7 days to restore full COC efficacy) with elimination of the next PFI if the 2 weeks of antibiotic use involved any of the last seven pills of a pack.

Long-term use of enzyme inducers

This applies chiefly to epileptic women and women being treated for tuberculosis. An alternative method of contraception is preferable, especially for those on rifampicin or rifabutin, whose adverse effects on efficacy of the COC are such that long-term users are strongly advised against it.

Relevant options that should *always first be discussed* are the injectable DMPA (with no special advice now needed to shorten the injection interval), an IUD, or the LNG-IUS.

Recommended regimen
If the combined pill is nevertheless chosen (see Table 22.4, the following guidelines are recommended:
- Prescribe an increased dose, usually 50–60 micrograms estrogen, by taking two tablets daily, and
- Advise using one of the placebo-free regimens described above. (This is particularly appropriate for epileptic women, since the frequency of attacks is often reduced by the maintenance of steady hormone levels.)

Table 22.4 Available combination oral contraceptives

Name	Progestin (mg)	Type of estrogen (mcg)
50 mcg estrogen		
Ogestrel, Oval	Norgestrel (0.5)	Ethinylestradiol (50)
Necon, Nelova, Norethin, Norinyl, Ortho-Novum 1/50	Norethindrone (1.0)	Mestranol (50)
Ovcon 50	Norethindrone (1.0)	Ethinylestradiol (50)
Norlestrin 1/50	Norethindrone acetate (1.0)	Ethinylestradiol (50)
Demulen 50, Zovia 1/50	Ethynodiol diacetate (1.0)	Ethinylestradiol (50)
<50 mcg estrogen plus monophasic		
Lo-Ovral, Low-Ogestrel	Norgestrel (0.3)	Ethinylestradiol (30)
Ovcon 35	Norethindrone (0.4)	Ethinylestradiol (35)
Desogen, Ortho-cept	Desogestrel (0.15)	Ethinylestradiol (30)
Levlen, Levora, Nordette	Levonorgestrel (0.15)	Ethinylestradiol (30)
Ortho-Cyclen	Norgestimate (0.25)	Ethinylestradiol (35)
Necon, Nelova, Norinyl, Norethrin, Ortho-Novum 1/35	Norethindrone (1.0)	Ethinylestradiol (35)
Lo-Ovral	Norgestrel (0.3)	Ethinylestradiol (30)
Brevicon, Modicon, Necon, Nelova 0.5/35	Norethindrone (0.5)	Ethinylestradiol (35)
Loestrin 1.5/30	Norethindrone acetate (1.5)	Ethinylestradiol (30)
Alesse, Levlite 0.1/20	Levonorgestrel (0.1)	Ethinylestradiol (20)

Table 22.4 (Contd.)

Name	Progestin (mg)	Type of estrogen (mcg)
Seasonale 15/30	Levonorgestrel (0.15)	Ethinylestradiol (30)
Loestrin 1/20	Norethindrone acetate (1.0)	Ethinylestradiol (20)
Demulen, Zovia 1/35	Ethynodiol diacetate (1.0)	Ethinylestradiol (35)
<50 mcg estrogen plus multiphasic		
Ortho-Novum 7/7/7	Norethindrone (0.5, 0.75, 1.0)	Ethinylestradiol (35, 35, 35)
Tri-Levlen, Triphasil, Trivora	Levonorgestrel (0.05, 0.075, 0.125)	Ethinylestradiol (30, 40, 30)
Jenest	Norethindrone (0.5, 1.0)	Ethinylestradiol (35, 35)
Necon, Nelova, Ortho-Novum 10/11	Norethindrone (0.5, 1.0)	Ethinylestradiol (35, 35)
Ortho Tri-Cyclen	Norgestimate (0.18, 0.215, 0.250)	Ethinylestradiol (35, 35, 35)
Tri-Norinyl	Norethindrone (0.5, 1.0, 0.5)	Ethinylestradiol (35, 35)
Estrostep	Norethindrone acetate (1.0, 1.0, 1.0)	Ethinylestradiol (20, 30, 35)
Mircette	Desogestrel (0.15)	Ethinylestradiol (0.02, 0.01)
Other		
Yasmin	Drospirenone (3)	Ethinylestradiol (30)

Counseling and ongoing supervision

Starting the COC
- Full personal and family history
- Individual teaching
- 21-day combined pill is started on the Sunday after the period without additional contraception.
- In nonlactating women, 21-day or 28-day brands may be started 21 days after vaginal delivery, provided there are no puerperal complications. Additional contraceptive measures should be taken for 7 days.
- After a first-trimester termination, an oral contraceptive can be started immediately (see Table 22.4).

Take-home messages for a new pill taker
- The pill only works if you take it correctly. If you do, each new pack will always start on the same day of the week.
- Even if bleeding, such as a menstrual period, occurs (BTB), continue to take the pill—call for advice if necessary. Nausea is another common early symptom. Both usually settle as your body gets used to the pill.
- *Never be a late restarter* of your pill. Even if your period (withdrawal bleed) has not stopped yet, never start your next packet late.
- Intercourse during the 7 days after any packet is taken is only safe if you actually go on to the next pack. Otherwise, if you decide to stop the method, you must start using condoms after the last pill in the pack.
- For instructions on what to do if any pill(s) are taken >24 hours late, see the previous bullets.
- Other things that may stop the pill from working include vomiting and some drugs (always mention to your provider that you are on the pill).
- You can avoid bleeding on holidays, etc. by running packs together. (Discuss this with whoever provides your pills if you want to continue missing menstrual periods long term.)
- The pill does not protect against *Chlamydia* and other sexually transmitted diseases (STDs). Whenever in doubt, especially with a new partner, use a condom as well.

Second choice of pill brand
Some women react unpredictably, and it is a false expectation that any single pill will suit all women.

Bleeding side effects
Given the model shown in Fig. 22.3 by the variability of blood levels and BTB risk, prescribers should try to identify the lowest dose for each woman that does not cause BTB. Even if BTB occurs, provided there is ongoing good compliance with pill taking, extra contraception (e.g., with condoms) does not need to be advised.

The objective is that each woman receive the least long-term metabolic impact that her uterus will allow, i.e., the lowest dose of contraceptive steroids that is just, but only just, above her bleeding threshold.

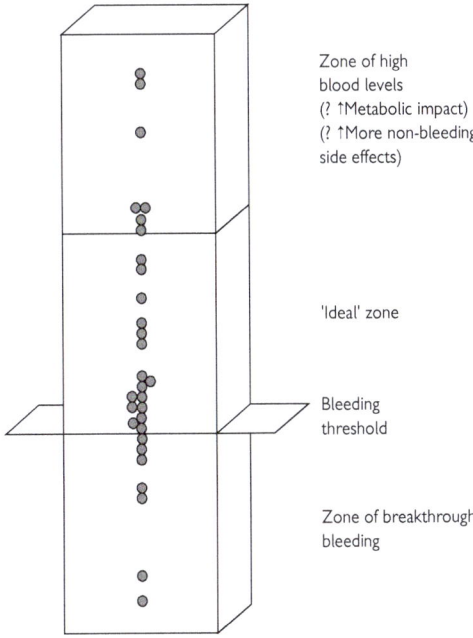

Figure 22.3 Schematic representation of the marked individual variations in blood levels of contraceptive steroids.

If BTB does occur and is unacceptable or persists beyond two cycles, a different or higher-dose brand should be tried (see Table 22.4).
The checklist for abnormal bleeding, presented in Box 22.1, is modified from Sapire.[1]

Second choice if there are nonbleeding side effects

When symptoms occur, it is generally bad practice to give further prescriptions to control them without changing the COC—such as diuretics for weight gain or antidepressants for mood symptoms.

There are two main preferred, if empirical, courses of action:
- Decrease the dose of either hormone, if possible (estrogen can be eliminated by a trial of a POP), or
- Change to a different progestogen.

---

[1] Sapire KE (1990). *Contraception and Sexuality in Health and Disease*. New York: McGraw-Hill.

Box 22.1 Checklist for abnormal bleeding in a pill user

- DISEASE. Consider examining the cervix (it is not unknown for bleeding from an invasive cancer to be wrongly attributed, and any bloodstained discharge should always trigger the thought "chlamydia?").
- DISORDERS of PREGNANCY that cause bleeding (e.g., retained products if the COC was started after a recent termination of pregnancy)
- DEFAULT. BTB may be triggered 2 or 3 days after missed pills and may be persistent thereafter.
- DRUGS, primarily enzyme inducers (see text). Cigarettes are also drugs in this context: BTB is statistically more common among smokers.
- Diarrhea and/or VOMITING. Diarrhea alone has to be exceptionally severe to impair absorption significantly.
- DISTURBANCES of ABSORPTION, for example, after bowel disease or resection
- DURATION of USE that is too short, i.e., assessment is too early (minimal BTB that is tolerable for longer may then cease after 3 months' use of any new formulation). The opposite possibility may apply during use of a continuous OC, namely that the duration of continuous use has been too long for the woman's endometrium to be sustained, in which case a bleeding–triggered 4- to 7-day break may be taken.
- DOSE. After the above factors have been excluded, it is possible to increase the progestogen component or the estrogen if a 20 microgram COC is in use, or try a different progestogen.

Which second choice of pill? Relative estrogen excess

Symptoms

- Nausea
- Dizziness
- Cyclical weight gain (fluid), bloating—Yasmin® is also worth a try here, given the antimineralocorticoid activity of DSP.
- Vaginal discharge (no infection)
- Some cases of breast enlargement or pain
- Some cases of lost libido without depression, especially if taking an antiandrogen (Yasmin® or Dianette®)

Conditions

- Benign breast disease
- Fibroids
- Endometriosis

Treat these conditions with a relatively progestogen-dominant COC, such as Microgynon 30®. Loestrin 20® is an estrogen-deficient option.

Which second choice of pill? Relative progestogen excess

Symptoms
- Dryness of vagina
- Some cases of sustained weight gain—although there is actually no good evidence that modern COCs cause the weight gain for which they are often blamed
- Depression, lassitude
- Depressed mood ± associated loss of libido
- Breast tenderness

Conditions
- Acne, seborrhea
- Hirsutism

Treat these conditions with an estrogen-dominant COC or, in moderately severe cases of acne or hirsutism, with Yasmin® (see text). (Exercise caution when using Yasmin®, because estrogen dominance may correlate with a slightly higher risk of VTE, especially with obesity [Table 22.2]).

More about Yasmin®

- Acne, seborrhea, and sometimes hirsutism may be benefited by any of the COCs. Yasmin® is a monophasic COC containing 3 mg DSP and 30 micrograms EE. DSP differs from other progestogens in COCs in that
- It acts as an antiandrogen when used in the treatment of moderately severe acne and PCOS.
- It has diuretic properties due to antimineralocorticoid activity.

Yasmin® is welcomed as a new choice for appropriate women, for example:

- It is a clear indication for estrogen/antiandrogen therapy, such as moderately severe acne.
- It is a useful second choice for empirical control of minor side effects, particularly those associated with fluid retention such as bloating and cyclical breast enlargement. It seems to be of value for women with the premenstrual syndrome, whether in their normal cycle or occurring on another COC, in which case continuous use or tri-cycling is preferable.

Stopping COCs

Listed here are the (only) reasons for discontinuing COCs immediately or soon. These reasons should be understood by all well-counseled women from their first visit on.

The worst implications of these symptoms are pill-related thrombotic or embolic catastrophes in the making, or onset of migraine with aura. Often there is another explanation; if so, the COC may be restarted.

The COC containing EE should be stopped, but any progestogen-only method could be started immediately pending diagnosis.

Symptoms for which COCs should be stopped immediately, pending investigation and treatment

- Unusual or severe and very prolonged headache
- Diagnosis of aura (see p. 208), usually involving loss of part or all of the field of vision on one side
- Loss of sight in one eye (unrelated to migraine)
- Disturbance of speech (nominal dysphasia in migraine with aura)
- Numbness, severe paresthesia, or weakness on one side of the body, e.g., one arm, side of the tongue; any symptom suggesting cerebral ischemia or TIA
- A severe unexplained fainting attack or severe acute vertigo or ataxia
- Focal epilepsy
- Painful swelling in the calf
- Pain in the chest, especially pleuritic pain
- Breathlessness or cough with blood-stained sputum
- Severe abdominal pain
- Immobilization, e.g.,
- After most lower limb fractures or
- *Major* surgery or
- Leg surgery

For all these, stop COC use and consider heparin treatment. If an elective procedure is planned and the pill stopped >2 weeks ahead (4 weeks preferable), anticoagulation may be unnecessary.

Other reasons for early discontinuation
- Acute jaundice
- BP >160/>95 mmHg (either figure) on repeated measurement
- Severe skin rash (e.g., erythema multiforme)
- Detection of a significant new risk factor, e.g., onset of severe SLE, first diagnosis of breast cancer

Other combined methods

Contraception patch (Ortho Evra)

The patch contains a combination of estrogen and progestin. A new patch is applied weekly and can be stopped for 1 week for induction of menses or used in a continuous fashion.

Given the lack of "first-pass" effect seen with oral agents on the liver, it was speculated that the risk of DVT would be decreased; however, there are reports of increased risk due to the sustained release and higher continuous levels of estrogen.

The contraception path should not be considered safer but may be a favorable alterative to those who do not like oral medication or those with significant intestinal disease.

Vaginal ring (NuvaRing)

The vaginal contraceptive ring contains estrogen and progestin, as does a pill or patch.

The ring is placed in the vagina and, as with the patch, continuously releases estrogen and progesterone, which is absorbed by the vagina.

It is suited for those who do not wish to take oral medication and do not want to have a patch visible.

Pill follow-up

Primarily this entails two items to be monitored:
- BP
- Headaches, especially migraine

Blood pressure
- BP is recorded before COCs are started and checked after 3 months (1 month in a high-risk case) and subsequently at intervals of 6 months.
- After a minimum of 15 months, if there is no rise between successive measurements, the interval can reasonably be increased to annually in women without risk factors (with a clear understanding that they may return for advice sooner, as desired).
- COCs should always be stopped altogether if BP exceeds 160/95 mmHg on repeated measurements.

Headaches

Neglecting to ask about a COC taker's headaches at the regular pill follow-up visit would be a serious omission.

Screening

Breast and bimanual pelvic examinations or monitoring blood tests have no relevance to pill follow-up.

Congenital abnormalities and fertility issues

Even with exposure during organogenesis, meta-analyses of the major studies fail to show an increased risk. If present, it must be very small.

Used prior to the conception cycle, there is no good evidence for any adverse effects of COCs on the fetus.

These meta-analyses are of no value, as there is no evidence that COCs can cause any permanent loss of fertility.

Summary

The first visit for prescription of COCs is by far the most important one and should never be rushed.

The long-acting reversible contraceptives (LARCs), long-term and "forgettable" contraceptive options, should always be included in the discussion, despite the woman's request for the method that she is most familiar with (most probably the pill).

Thereafter, there are really only three key components to COC monitoring during follow-up:
- BP
- Headaches
- Identification and management of any new risk factors, diseases, or side effects

Chapter 23

The progestogen-only pill (POP)

Mechanism of action and maintenance of effectiveness 224
Risks and disadvantages 225
Advantages and indications 226
Problems and contraindications 227
Counseling and ongoing supervision 228

Mechanism of action and maintenance of effectiveness

Fertile ovulation is prevented in 50–60% of cycles.

In the remainder there is reliance mainly on *progestogenic interference with mucus penetrability*. This barrier effect is readily lost, so each tablet daily must be taken within 3 hours of the same regular time.

Effectiveness

There is a failure rate of 3.1 per 100 woman-years between the ages 25 and 29, but this improves to 1.0 at 35–39 years of age and can be as low as 0.3 for women >40 years of age.

Missed pills

After missing a POP for >3 hours, the woman should do the following:
- Take that day's pill immediately and the next one on time.
- Use added precautions for the next 2 days.

If there has already been intercourse without added protection between the time of first potential loss of the mucus effect and through to its restoration by 48 hours, immediate emergency contraception (EC) with levonorgestrel (LNG) (see below) is also advised. The next POP should be taken on time.

What action is necessary with POP use during full lactation?

Here there is established anovulation. So only the two bullets under "Missed pills" would apply, and EC would be unnecessary in most cases. Pending more data, EC could be given on a fail-safe basis for omissions of more than one pill, i.e., beyond 24 hours.

More about lactation and the POP

Even without the POP there is only ~2% conception risk if all of the following apply:
- Amenorrhea, since the lochia ceased
- Full lactation—the baby's nutrition is effectively all from its mother
- Baby not yet 6 months old

This is why on any POP during full lactation, postcoital contraception would very rarely be indicated for missed POPs. But because breastfeeding varies in its intensity, if a tablet is taken 3 hours late, it is still common to advise using additional precautions during the next two tablet-taking days.

What dose goes to the baby?

During lactation, with all POPs the dose to the infant is believed to be harmless; this aspect must always be discussed with the patient. The quantity is the equivalent of one POP in 2 years, considerably less than the progesterone of cow's milk found in formula feeds.

If EC is required (rarely, see above) by a breastfeeding mother, for just 24 hours she may wish to express and discard her breast milk, although even then there is no evidence that this higher LNG dose would cause her baby any harm.

Drug interactions

Broad-spectrum antibiotics
These do not interfere with the effectiveness of POPs or any progestogen-only method.

Enzyme inducers
Another highly effective contraceptive method is advised during use of liver enzyme inducers such as rifampicin or carbamazepine and, as necessary, for 4 weeks or more thereafter (see Chapter 22).

Long-term treatment with enzyme inducers should lead one to reconsider an alternate contraceptive, but if a suitable alternative contraceptive is not identified and the couple does not wish to use condoms indefinitely, taking two tablets daily is an option.

Risks and disadvantages

Being ethinylestradiol (EE)-free, these are exceptionally safe products. There are negligible changes to most metabolic variables. There is no proven causative link
- with any tumor
- with venous or (less certainly) arterial disease

Side effects

The main side effect of POPs is irregular bleeding.

The irregularity can include oligomenorrhea. FSH is not completely suppressed even during the amenorrhea, which is mainly caused by LH suppression. There is therefore enough follicular activity at the ovary to maintain adequate mid-follicular phase estrogen levels.

Pending more data, this means there is *not* the concern about bone density reduction that persists with DMPA (see p. 235).

Advantages and indications

The indications for POP use are listed in Box 23.1.

> **Box 23.1 Indications for POP use**
> - Lactation, where the combination even with ordinary POPs is extra effective, as good as the COC would be in non-breastfeeders
> - Side effects with or recognized contraindications to the combined pill, particularly when the effects are estrogen related. As EE-free products do not appear to affect blood-clotting mechanisms significantly, POPs may be used by women with a definite past history of venous thromboembolism (VTE) and a whole range of disorders predisposing to arterial or venous disease. Good counseling and record keeping are essential.
> - Sickle cell disease, severe structural heart disease, pulmonary hypertension
> - Smokers >35 years of age
> - Hypertension, whether COC related or not, controlled on treatment
> - Migraine, including varieties with aura (the woman may well continue to suffer migraines, but the fear of an EE-promoted thrombotic stroke is eliminated). POP use is at the woman's choice.

Problems and contraindications

Absolute contraindications for POP and use
These are far fewer than for the COCs (see also Box 23.2 and Box 23.3).
- Any serious adverse effect of COCs not certainly related solely to the estrogen (e.g., liver adenoma or cancer)
- Breast cancer
- Acute porphyria, if history of an actual attack is triggered by hormones (progestogens and estrogens are believed capable of precipitating these)
- Undiagnosed genital tract bleeding
- Actual or possible pregnancy
- Hypersensitivity to any component

Box 23.2 Strong relative contraindications for POP use
- Past severe arterial diseases or current exceptionally high risk thereof
- Sex steroid–dependent cancer, including breast cancer, even when in complete remission, alters the recurrence risk (either way).
- Recent trophoblastic disease until hCG is undetectable in blood and in urine
- Enzyme inducers (POPs can be taken, but another method such as an IUD or LNG-IUS would be preferable)
- Acute porphyria, latent or with no hormone-triggered previous attack (along with caution, forewarning or monitoring); the POP is fully usable in all nonacute porphyrias.
- Past symptomatic (painful) functional ovarian cysts. But a persistent cyst or follicles that are commonly detected on routine ultrasonography can be disregarded if they caused no symptoms.
- Previous treatment for ectopic pregnancy; however, this is an indication for POP! The risk of ectopic pregnancy is actually reduced among POP users. But it can be reduced still further by using methods that markedly reduce fertilization rates (such as the COC, DMPA).

Box 23.3 Relative contraindications for POP and use
- Past VTE or severe risk factors for VTE—often an indication (see previous section)
- Risk factors for arterial disease; more than one risk factor can be present, in contrast to COCs
- Current liver disorder—even if there is persistent biochemical change
- Most other chronic severe systemic diseases

Counseling and ongoing supervision

The starting routines are summarized in Table 23.1.

A crucial aspect of counseling is how not to forget pill-taking, given the 3-hour time window. Mobile phone alarms and text messaging may be invaluable for complete adherence.

Frequent or prolonged menstrual bleeding

This is the main nuisance side effect. With advance warning, it may be tolerated.

Amenorrhea

Except during full lactation, prolonged spells of amenorrhoea occur most often in older women. Once pregnancy is excluded, the amenorrhea must be the result of anovulation and thus signifies very high efficacy.

Nonbleeding side effects

These are rare with POPs, apart from the complaint of the following:
- *Breast tenderness*. Although common, this is usually transient.
- *Functional cysts* or luteinized unruptured follicles are also not uncommon; however, most are symptomless and pelvic pain on one or the other side is relatively unusual.

Table 23.1 Starting routine for POPs

Condition before start	Start when?	Extra precautions
Menstruation	Day 1 of period	No
	Day 2 or later	7 days
	Any time in cycle ("quick start")	7 days[1]
Postpartum		
No lactation	Usually day 21	No
Lactation	Day 21—may be later if 100% lactation	No
After induced abortion or miscarriage	Same day	No
After COCs	Instant switch	No
Amenorrhea (e.g., postpartum)	Any time[2]	7 days

[1] Can start any day in selected cases if the prescriber is satisfied that there has been no conception risk on the starting day.

[2] If prescriber is confident that no blastocyst or sperm is already in the upper genital tract (see 📖 p. 276).

Monitoring

The BP of POP takers is checked initially, but thereafter, if it is still normal at the 3-month follow-up visit, it really does not need to be checked more often than for other women.

When raised during COC use, it usually reverts to normal on POPs.

Return of fertility after POPs

This is rapid: clinically, from the user's point of view, fertility after stopping must be assumed to be immediate.

Menopause

Establishing ovarian failure at menopause is less important than with the COC, since all the POPs are safe enough products to continue using well into the late 50s. Hence, first switching to any POP from the COC can be a reassuring way to manage the often difficult transition out of the reproductive years.

If there is amenorrhea in women on the POP who are above the age of 50, a high blood FSH measurement (>30 IU/L) suggests ovarian failure. Two high values 6 weeks apart, especially if there are vasomotor symptoms, would make the likelihood of a later ovulation very low.

Should the FSH be found to be low, however, this suggests continuing ovarian function and, if the POP is not simply continued, there may be need for an additional contraceptive.

Chapter 24

Injectables

Introduction *232*
Mechanism of action and effectiveness *233*
Indications *234*
Advantages *234*
Problems and disadvantages *235*
Contraindications *237*
Counseling and ongoing supervision *238*

Introduction

Background

In the United States, the only injectable contraceptive currently licensed for long-term use is depot medroxyprogesterone acetate (DMPA).

WHO data indicate that DMPA users have a reduced risk of cancer, with no overall increased risk of cancers of the breast, ovary, or cervix and a 5-fold reduction in the risk of carcinoma of the endometrium (relative risk 0.2).

Administration

There are two injectable agents available:
- DMPA 150 mg every 12 weeks

DMPA is generally given by deep IM injection within the first 5 days of the menstrual cycle. Injections may also be given beyond day 5, along with 7 days' added precautions if it is near certain that a conception risk has not been taken. In the United States, the injection sites are usually in the right upper quadrant of either buttock; the area should not be massaged.
- *Subcutaneous DMPA* is not yet available in the United States. It delivers a lower dose (104 mg) of medroxyprogesterone acetate (MPA) than that of standard Depo-Provera® for a similar duration of effectiveness.

Mechanism of action and effectiveness

DMPA is one of the most effective among reversible contraceptive methods. It has a "perfect-use" failure rate of 0.3% and a "typical-use" rate of 3% in the first year of use.

DMPA functions primarily by causing anovulation, with effects on the cervical mucus that are similar to those of the combined oral contraceptive (COC), as back-up.

Potential drug interactions

The liver ordinarily clears the blood, achieving complete clearance of the drug and, as enzyme inducers cannot increase clearance beyond 100%, there is no requirement to shorten the injection interval. This applies even to users of the most powerful enzyme inducers, rifampicin and rifabutin.

Starting routines

See Box 24.1 for timing of the first injection.

◆ Overdue injections of DMPA with continuing sexual intercourse

- From day 85 to 91 (13th week): injection plus condoms or the equivalent to be used during the next 7 days
- From day 92 to 98 (14th week): injection plus emergency contraception (EC) by hormone (or, more rarely, copper IUD) as appropriate, plus condoms for 7 days

Box 24.1 Timing of the first injection of DMPA

- In menstruating women, the first injection should ideally be given on day 1 but can be up to day 5 of the cycle. If given later than day 5 (including *much* later if abstinence is believably claimed to that day), advise 7 days' use of extra precautions.
- If a woman is on a COC or POP or up to the day of injection, the injection can normally be given at any time, with no added precautions.
- Postpartum (when the woman is not breastfeeding) or after a second-trimester abortion, the first injection should normally be at about day 21 and, if later, along with added precautions for 7 days. If the injection is later and the woman is still amenorrhoeic, pregnancy risk must be excluded. Earlier use can lead to prolonged heavy bleeding but is sometimes clinically justified.
- During lactation, if chosen, DMPA is best given at 6 weeks. Lactation is *not* inhibited and the dose to the infant is small and believed to be entirely harmless.
- After miscarriage or a first-trimester abortion, injection should be given on the same day (or after expulsion of fetus if a medical procedure). If the injection is given beyond the 7th day, advise 7 days of extra precautions.

- Beyond day 98, end of 14th week:
- The next injection is best postponed, usually for a few days.
- If possible, reach agreement with the woman that she will either abstain from intercourse or use condoms with greater care than ever before, UNTIL there has been both a total of 14 days since the last sexual exposure and a sensitive pregnancy test showing negative.
- If a sensitive (20–25 IU/L) pregnancy test is then negative, the chances of conception are negligible and the next dose can be given along with the usual advice for a further 7 days of added contraception, e.g., with condoms. No EC would then be needed, but a follow-up pregnancy test in a further 2 weeks might be wise.
- If the woman is not prepared to abstain from intercourse or to use condoms for the necessary number of days to reach 14 since her last sex, a useful compromise is to provide the progestogen-only pill (POP) for that time and then proceed as above. The teratogenic risks to a fetus exposed to the POP (and DMPA) have been established as being very low.

In all circumstances, counsel the woman about possible failure and the need for a check pregnancy test if there is doubt.

Indications

The main indications are as follows:
- The woman's desire for a highly effective method that is independent of intercourse and unaffected by enzyme inducers
- When other options are contraindicated or disliked
- A past history of ectopic pregnancy or, like all other progestogen-only methods, of thrombosis (see earlier comments on the POP, p. 226), e.g., for effective contraception while waiting for major surgery.

DMPA is also beneficial in:
- Endometriosis
- Past symptomatic functional cysts
- Other menstrual disorders

Advantages

DMPA has the following advantages:
- Obvious contraceptive benefits (effective, "forgettable")
- Most of the noncontraceptive benefits of the COC that were described earlier (see p. 195), including protection against pelvic infection and endometrial cancer
- Even greater safety, with respect to mortality and serious morbidity, than the COC. This should strongly counterbalance any concerns about bone density, described in the next section (p. 235).

Problems and disadvantages

Metabolic changes are minimal, aside from some evidence of reduction in high-density lipoprotein (HDL) cholesterol.

The main problems are as follows:
- Irregular, sometimes prolonged bleeding
- Amenorrhea and potential hypoestrogenism
- Impossibility of reversal of the effect of a dose (for at least 3 months, sometimes longer). It is necessary to mention this fact in advance.
- Delayed return of fertility—also something the patient should be warned of (see below).
- Weight gain (which can be marked in some cases)
- Some concern about reduced bone density, which is probably exaggerated

Menstrual abnormalities

These are obstacles to any large increase in the method's popularity.

In the management of frequent or prolonged bleeding:
- First, always exclude a non-DMPA-related cause (see 📖 p. 218).
- It has a better prognosis than that with implants, being usually an early problem that is generally followed by amenorrhea after 3–6 months.
- If it does not resolve, the next injection may be given early (but not less than 4 weeks since the last dose).

However, clinical experience suggests that giving additional estrogen is more successful, though not proven in trials. The rationale is to provide estrogen cyclically to produce some "pharmacological curettages," i.e., withdrawal bleeds designed to shed the existing endometrium that is bleeding in an unacceptable way, in hopes that a "better" endometrium will be developed post-treatment.

The plan should be explained to the woman, who should also understand that it is not guaranteed to work. The treatment options are as follows:
- 🔑 EE 30 mcg (often as an OC). It is given daily for 21 days, for up to three cycles. Courses may be repeated if an acceptable bleeding pattern does not follow.
- 🔑 If the woman has a contraindication to EE, an alternative that has been effective short term is doxycycline 100 mg bid for 5 days.

Amenorrhea occurs in most long-term users and is usually acceptable, after appropriate counseling.

Bone density

After >20 years of research but no RCTs or adequate comparative studies, there remains uncertainty—not about the low-follicular-phase estradiols that are found in many DMPA users but about their implications for bone health.

We know that mean bone density is lower in DMPA users than that in controls in cross-sectional comparisons, including among women above age 45. This finding is unconnected to the bleeding pattern (it may or may not occur in women experiencing either amenorrhea or irregular bleeding).

Bone density increases upon discontinuation (suggestive of a real effect, but also very reassuring for reversibility).

From limited evidence, there is decreased bone mineral density in adolescent DMPA users compared with that in controls using implants (or COCs). This has raised concern that *peak bone mass* that is fully developed by age 25 might be lower in DMPA users.

Yet women using DMPA long term who were examined after menopause and lifetime never-users have not been shown to differ in bone density. This suggests recovery of bone mass after stopping DMPA use.

An excess of limb or vertebral fractures has never been shown in long-term DMPA users.

How long to use DMPA?

Careful re-evaluation of risks and benefits is required in all those who wish to continue use for more than 2 years (see Boxes 24.2 and 24.3).

Box 24.2 Cautions in use of DMPA

- If there is known osteopenia or if strong risk factors exist, namely:
- Long-term corticosteroid treatment
- Secondary amenorrhea due to anorexia nervosa or marathon running
- A significant malabsorption syndrome

For all these, DMPA is contraindicated unless a bone scan shows no osteopenia, the risk factor has ceased, and the young woman has been obtaining either natural estrogen during normal cycling or EE through the COC.

Under age 19, given the concern that DMPA may prevent achievement of peak bone mass, it may be used only after other methods have been discussed and are found to be unsuitable or unacceptable.

Box 24.3 DMPA use for all other women

- DMPA remains a highly effective, safe, and "forgettable" method, usable by almost any woman in the childbearing years.
- Every 2 years there should be a regular formal discussion and reassessment of alternatives, but without blood tests or any imaging. These (e.g., bone density scanning) would only be appropriate if indicated for that particular woman on specific clinical grounds.
- Many women will therefore choose to switch from DMPA to another long-acting method, e.g., to Implanon®, IUD or IUS, after 2, 4, 6 or 8 years.
- But if the woman wishes to use DMPA for a longer period of time, even much longer, it is appropriate, after counseling.

Remember, when all is said and done, DMPA is clearly safer than the EE-containing COC!

Are there similar bone density concerns with long-term use of Implanon® or the POP?

No, the data are reassuring so far about both estradiol and bone density: in comparative 2-year studies, data for both remained similar to those for copper IUD users.

Contraindications

Absolute contraindications for DMPA

- Past severe arterial disease or current very high risk thereof (because of the evidence of low estrogen levels being coupled with reports of lowered HDL cholesterol)
- Current osteopenia or severe risk factor(s) for osteoporosis, including chronic corticosteroid treatment (>5 mg per day)
- Any serious adverse effect of COCs not related solely to the estrogen (e.g., liver adenoma or cancer)
- Breast cancer
- Acute porphyria, even if latent—no history of actual attack (progestogens and estrogens are believed capable of precipitating these, and the injection is not removable)
- Undiagnosed genital tract bleeding
- Actual or possible pregnancy
- Hypersensitivity to any component

Relative contraindications for DMPA

- Short-term steroid treatment, recovered anorexia nervosa with normal menstrual cycling: see Box 24.2.
- Age <18 years
- Active liver disease with abnormal liver function tests
- Recent trophoblastic disease, until hCG is undetectable in blood as well as urine.
- DMPA is usable in all non-acute porphyrias.
- Sex steroid–dependent cancer, including breast cancer, in complete remission
- Unacceptability of menstrual irregularities, especially when related to cultural and religious taboos, whether associated with bleeding or amenorrhea.
- Obesity, although further weight gain is not inevitable (see next section)
- Past severe endogenous depression
- Planning a pregnancy in the near future (see next section)

Counseling and ongoing supervision

Four practical points must always be made to prospective users:
1. The effects, whether wanted (contraceptive) or unwanted, are *not* reversible for the duration of the injection: this fact is unique among current contraceptives.
2. After the last dose, conception is commonly delayed, with a median delay of 9 months, which is only 6 months after cessation of the method. But in some individuals it could be well over 1 year.
3. Weight gain is probable because of increased appetite, so it is useful (and can really work) to advise a pre-emptive plan to start getting extra exercise as well as watching diet.
4. Irregular, sometimes prolonged bleeding may be a problem, but the outlook is good, as it is usually followed after a few months by amenorrhea, which (it should be explained) is not a problem.

Follow-up

Apart from ensuring that the injections take place at the correct intervals, follow-up is primarily advisory and supportive.
- Prolonged or too frequent bleeding is managed as already described.
- BP is normally checked initially, but there is absolutely no need for it to be taken before each dose, as studies fail to show any hypertensive effect. An annual check is reasonable as well-woman care.

Chapter 25

Contraceptive implants

Introduction 240
Mechanism of action, administration, and effectiveness 241
Enzyme inducer drug (EID) treatment 242
Reversibility and removal problems 242
Indications 243
Advantages 243
Disadvantages and contraindications 244
Counseling and ongoing supervision 245

Chapter 25 Contraceptive implants

Introduction

Contraceptive implants contain a progestogen in a slow-release carrier, with two implants, or ethylene vinyl acetate (EVA) as Implanon®, a single rod (Fig. 25.1).

They are excellent examples of long-acting reversible contraceptives (LARCs) with the ideal "forgettable" default state yet rapid reversibility.

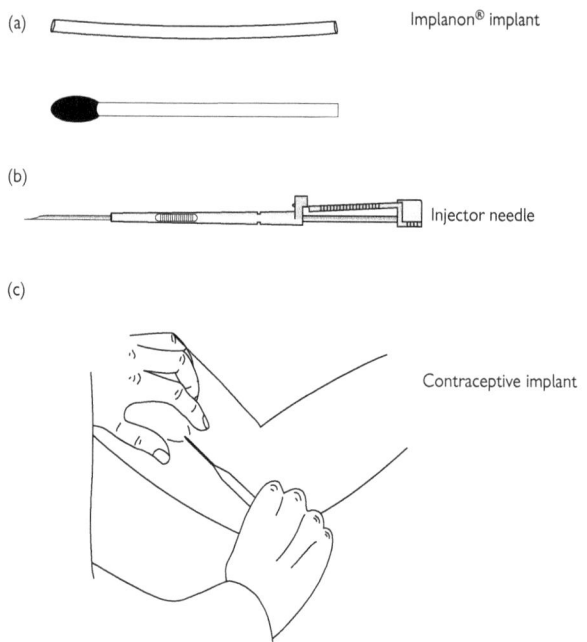

Figure 25.1 Implanon® contraceptive implant.

Mechanism of action, administration, and effectiveness

Implanon® works primarily by ovulation inhibition, supplemented mainly by the usual sperm-blocking mucus effect of progestogen.

It is a single 40-mm rod, just 2 mm in diameter, containing 68 mg of etonogestrel—the chief active metabolite of desogestrel. This is dispersed in an EVA matrix and covered by a 0.06-mm rate-limiting EVA membrane.

Clinically

The implant is inserted subdermally over the biceps medially in the upper arm, with local anesthesia, from a dedicated sterile preloaded applicator by means of a simple injection–withdrawal technique, aided by the blunt bevel of its cleverly shaped wide-bore needle.

It is inserted anterior to the groove between the triceps and biceps, well away from the neurovascular bundle. After an initial phase of several weeks of delivering higher blood levels, Implanon® delivers almost constant low daily levels of the hormone, for a recommended duration of use of 3 years.

Although this implant is much easier than Norplant® to insert or remove, specific (model arm plus live) training is essential and cannot be obtained from any book.

Implanon® had the unique distinction of a zero failure rate in the pre-marketing trials. The "perfect use" (i.e., typical use) failure rate is now estimated at 5 in 10,000.

In nearly all of the "failures" that have been reported, either the insertion was carried out during a conception cycle or there was a failure to insert.

Effect of body mass

Serum levels tend to be lower in heavier women. But given the high margin of efficacy subsequently, failures have not been attributed to BMI.

Clinically

This finding should *not* detract in the slightest from offering Implanon® to overweight women for whom the COC (or Evra®) has a high venous thromboembolism (VTE) risk.

Enzyme inducer drug (EID) treatment

The SPC states that hepatic enzyme inducers may lower the blood levels of etonogestrel.

Therefore, women on *short-term treatment* with any of these drugs are advised to use a barrier method in addition and (because reversal of enzyme induction always takes time) for 28 days thereafter.

During *long-term EID treatment*, Organon has only one recommendation: to transfer to a nonhormonal method with removal of the Implanon®. However, given that Implanon® blood levels are ordinarily considerably higher in the first 18 months, another option to be considered, on a "named patient" basis, is early replacement, at 12–18 months.

Another possibility, and probably more effective as well as cheaper for long-term users, is switching to either depot medroxyprogesterone acetate (DMPA) or the levonorgestrel intrauterine system (LNG-IUS). EID users do very well with either of these.

Reversibility and removal problems

Reversal is normally simple, with almost immediate effect:
- Under local anesthetic, apply digital pressure on the proximal end of the Implanon® and use a 2-mm incision over the distal end to deliver that end of the rod. Removal is completed by grasping it with forceps.
- Again (see p. 241), removal training is crucial, using the "model arm" and live under supervision.

Removal problems, including discomfort, can be minimized with good training in both the insertion and removal techniques.

Difficult removals correlate with initially too-deep insertion. Use careful technique particularly in thin or very muscular women with very little subcutaneous tissue. Insertion can easily permit a segment of the rod to enter the (biceps) muscle, with deep migration ensuing.

Specialized ultrasound techniques are required to localize "lost" Implanons®, and removal may need to be done under ultrasound control.

Indications

Being an anovulant, special indications include past ectopic pregnancy and a possibility of having menstrual disorders, although the outcome is not reliably beneficial (because of irregular bleeding, see below).

See Box 25.1 for timing of Implanon® insertion.

Advantages

- It provides efficacy and convenience: if the bleeding pattern is acceptable, the implant is a "forgettable" contraceptive.
- Long action with one treatment (3 years); high continuation rates
- Absence of the initial peak dose given orally to the liver
- Blood levels are low and steady, rather than fluctuating (as with the progestogen-only pill [POP]) or initially too high (as with injectables). This feature along with absence of the initial peak dose to the liver minimizes metabolic changes.
- It is estrogen-free, thus definitely usable if there is a history of VTE.
- Median systolic BP and diastolic BP were unchanged in trials for up to 4 years.
- The implant is rapidly reversible: after removal, serum etonogestrel levels were undetectable within 1 week. In terms of contraception, return of fertility must be assumed to be almost immediate during the first week.

Box 25.1 Timing of Implanon® insertion

- In the woman's natural cycle, day 1–5 is the usual timing of insertion. If done any later than day 5 (assuming no sexual exposure up to that day), recommend additional contraception for 7 days.
- If a woman is on a COC or POP or DMPA, the implant can normally be inserted any time, with no added precautions.
- *Clinical implications*: insertions only in the tiny natural-cycle window are a necessary logistic, and conception risk is a nightmare! A useful practical tip is to recommend use of an anovulant method (i.e., one of those in last bullet) at counseling for use until the Implanon® insertion has been carried out.
- Following delivery (not breastfeeding) or second-trimester abortion, insertion on about day 21 is recommended, or if later, with additional contraception for 7 days. If done later and the woman is still amenorrheic, pregnancy risk should be excluded.
- If the woman is breastfeeding, insert Implanon® on day 21–28; there is no need for added contraception for 7 days.
- Following first-trimester abortion, immediate insertion is best
  - On the day of surgically induced abortion or second part of a medical abortion, or
  - Up to 7 days later.
  - If >7 days later, an added method such as condoms is recommended for 7 days.

Disadvantages and contraindications

Contraindications are very similar to those for the POP, since like it but unlike DMPA, Implanon® is an anovulant yet is immediately reversible (and they both contain essentially the same progestogen).

Local adverse effects
- Infection of the site
- Expulsion
- Migration and difficult removal (see p. 242)
- Scarring

Absolute contraindications for Implanon®
- Any serious adverse effect of COCs not certainly related solely to the estrogen (e.g., liver adenoma or cancer)
- Breast cancer
- Acute porphyria with history of actual attack precipitated by hormones
- Known or suspected pregnancy
- Undiagnosed genital tract bleeding
- Hypersensitivity to any component
- Active VTE disorder (There is no evidence that Implanon® [like other progestogen-only methods] would increase VTE risk.)

Relative contraindications
- Acute porphyria, latent, with no previous attack (plus forewarning and monitoring); Implanon® is also usable in those with nonacute porphyrias.
- Current severe liver disorder with persistent biochemical change
- Recent trophoblastic disease until hCG is undetectable in the blood as well as urine, then category WHO 1
- Sex steroid–dependent cancer, including breast cancer, in complete remission (WHO advises 5 years). In all cases, approval from the relevant hospital consultant should be obtained and the woman's autonomy respected. Record that she understands that it is unknown whether progestogen alone in Implanon® alters the recurrence risk.
- Enzyme inducers—see p. 242. (But using another method such as an IUD or IUS would be preferable.)
- Past symptomatic functional ovarian cysts—these might recur with use of Implanon®, especially in the third year.

Relative contraindications (WHO 2)
- Past VTE or severe risk factors for VTE; clinically, this is often an indication, see Advantages.
- Risk factors for arterial disease; more than one risk factor can be present
- Current liver disorder (now) with normal biochemistry
- Most other chronic severe systemic diseases
- Unacceptability of irregular menstrual bleeding. This remains a problem with all progestogen-only methods, including Implanon®.

Counseling and ongoing supervision

Explain the likely changes to the bleeding pattern and the possibility of hormonal side effects (see below). This discussion should be accompanied by a good leaflet, such as the FPA one, and well documented.

No treatment-specific follow-up is necessary (including no need for BP checks). The SPC recommends one follow-up visit at 3 months.

Bleeding problems

In the premarketing RCT comparing Implanon® with the old 6-implant Norplant®, although amenorrhea was significantly more common with Implanon®, the combined rates for the more annoying "frequent bleeding and spotting" and "prolonged bleeding and spotting" were very similar.

Clinical management

After eliminating unrelated causes for the bleeding (p. 243):
- The best short-term treatment is cyclical estrogen therapy, an OC, as explained for DMPA (p. 235). The plan should be explained to the woman, who should also understand that it is not certain to work. Courses may be repeated if an acceptable bleeding pattern does not follow. Or:
- An alternative that was effective, though only short-term in a pilot study, is doxycycline 100 mg bid for 5 days. The mechanism is believed to be an effect on endometrial enzymes and is probably independent of treating any chlamydial endometritis. But one should test for chlamydia first, as is usual with irregular bleeding.

Minor side effects

Reported in order of frequency, the minor side effects are as follows:

- Acne (but this might also improve!)
- Headache
- Abdominal pain
- Breast pain
- "Dizziness"
- Mood changes (depression, emotional lability)
- Libido decrease
- Hair loss

Weight gain

In the RCT mentioned earlier, the mean body weight increase over 2 years was 2.6% with Implanon® and 2.9% with Norplant®, while, in a parallel study, similar users of an IUD showed weight increases of 2.4% over the same time period. Weight seems to be less of a problem than with DMPA, though some individuals do find their weight gain unacceptable.

Bone mineral density

Since Implanon® suppresses ovulation and does not supply any estrogen, the same questions that have arisen with DMPA arise over possible hypoestrogenism. However, it appears that like other POPs, the suppression of FSH levels with Implanon® is less complete, allowing adequate follicular-phase estrogen levels (i.e., usually not as low as the levels in DMPA users).

In a nonrandomized comparative study, no bone density changes or differences were detected in either 44 Implanon® users or 29 users of copper IUDs over 2 years, which is reassuring.

Chapter 26

Intrauterine contraception

Introduction *248*
Copper-bearing devices *249*
The levonorgestrel-releasing intrauterine system (LNG-IUS) *255*

Introduction

Intrauterine contraceptives are currently of two distinct types (Fig. 26.1):
- Copper intrauterine devices, abbreviated as IUDs, in which the copper ion (the actual contraceptive) is released from a band or wire on a plastic carrier;
- Levonorgestrel-releasing intrauterine system (LNG-IUS), which releases that progestogen.

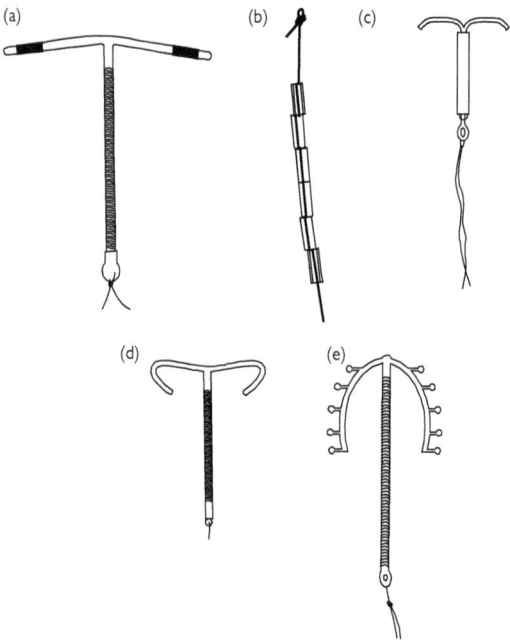

Figure 26.1 Illustration of some current IUDs (devices are not drawn to scale). (a) TT 380 Slimline®, (b) GyneFix®, (c) Mirena® (LNG-IUS), (d) Flexi-T 300®, (e) Multiload 375®.

Copper-bearing devices

Advantages of and indications for copper IUDs
- They are safe: the mortality rate is 1:500,000.
- They are effective:
- Immediately
- Postcoitally (but not true of the LNG-IUS)
- There is no link with coitus.
- There are no tablets to remember.
- Continuation rates are high and duration of use can exceed 10 years.
- They are reversible, and there is evidence that this is true even when IUDs have been removed for one of the recognized complications.

Mechanism of action
Appropriate studies indicate that copper IUDs operate primarily by preventing fertilization, the copper ion being toxic to sperm. When put in postcoitally, they can also act to block implantation.

However, when IUDs are in situ long term, this seems to be a rarely needed secondary or back-up mechanism.

Clinical implication
- Use an additional contraceptive method from 7 days before planned device removal, or if this has not been the case.
- Postpone removal until the next menses.

If a device must be removed earlier, hormonal postcoital contraception may be indicated.

Important influence of age on effectiveness
Copper IUDs are much more effective in older women, largely because of the women's declining fertility.

Over the age of 30 there is also a reduction in rates of expulsion and of pelvic inflammatory disease (PID). PID is not believed to be the result of the older uterus resisting infection; rather, the older women is generally less exposed to risk of infection (whether through her own lifestyle or that of her only partner).

Advantages of the banded IUDs
- Most IUD complications can be insertion related
- Most IUD complication are reduced in frequency with duration of use.

What if the woman is nulliparous?
Nulliparity per se is not a contraindication for this method. In a mutually monogamous relationship, especially above age 35, it should be seen as an accepted method.

Main problems and disadvantages of copper IUDs
The main medical problems are listed in Box 26.1. This is actually a remarkably short list compared with that for hormonal methods.

Box 26.1 Problems and disadvantages of copper IUDs

1. Intrauterine pregnancy, hence its risk including miscarriage
2. Extrauterine pregnancy is prevented less well than intrauterine, though the absolute risk is actually reduced in population terms.
3. Expulsion, hence the risk of pregnancy or miscarriage
4. Perforation
   - Risks to bowel and bladder
   - Risks of pregnancy
5. Pelvic infection—as with point 2, the IUD is *not* causative
6. Malpositioning (which predisposes to points 1, 3, and 7)
7. Pain
8. Bleeding
   - Increased amount
   - Increased duration

Pain and bleeding in IUD users signify a potentially dangerous condition, until proved otherwise.

All of the first six problems need to be excluded as diagnoses before pain and bleeding are ascribed to being side effects of this method.

In situ conception

If the woman wishes to go on to full-term pregnancy, after a pelvic ultrasound scan demonstrates an intrauterine pregnancy, the device should normally be removed.
- Spontaneous abortion was 55%, dropping to 20% if the device was removed.

Other clinical points
- If the woman is going to have a termination of her pregnancy, her IUD (or IUS) can be removed at the planned surgery; but it is safest to remove it before any medical abortion.
- If the threads are already missing when she is seen and other causes are excluded, aided by an ultrasound scan (see below), the pregnancy is at increased risk of the following:
- Second-trimester abortion (which could be infected)
- Antepartum hemorrhage
- Premature labor
- If the woman goes on to full term, it is essential to identify clearly the device in the products of conception. If it is not found, a postpartum X-ray should be arranged in case the device is embedded or malpositioned, or has perforated.

There have been many medicolegal cases when this was not done, leading to
- Problems from an undiagnosed perforation or
- Unnecessary tests and treatments for "infertility" when a much earlier malpositioned device with no visible threads had been left in situ.

IUDs with "lost threads"

The woman with "lost threads" is already pregnant until proven otherwise (moreover, even then she is probably unprotected and at risk of becoming pregnant).

Six possible causes of "lost threads" are listed in Table 26.1.

Diagnosis and management of this condition may involve the following:
- First, ascertaining if the threads are in fact present: they may be short and drawn up into the canal.
- Pregnancy testing
- Imaging by ultrasound, sometimes also X-ray
- Use of special extractors and forceps under local anesthetic
- Operative laparoscopy under general anesthetic

The later stages of this progression should be after referral to a specialist.

More about perforation

A general estimated risk of perforation for all IUDs is ~1 per 1000 insertions, but the exact rate (like for expulsion) depends much less on the IUD design than on the skill of the clinician.

Perforated devices should now almost always be removable at laparoscopy.

Pelvic inflammatory disease and IUDs—what is the truth?

IUDs, intrinsically, cannot be the cause of the PID that occurs in IUD users. Otherwise, in China (with a vanishingly low incidence of PID) there would have been at least one reported case among the 4301 IUD insertions in the WHO database presented in Fig. 26.2.

The greatest risk is during the first 20 days, most probably caused by pre-existing sexually transmitted disease (STDs). Risk thereafter, as with preinsertion, relates to the background STI risk.

Therefore, the evidence-based policy should be that elective IUD insertions and reinsertions should always occur through a cervix that has been established to be pathogen-free, thus effectively eliminating the postinsertion infections listed in Fig. 26.2.

Table 26.1 possible causes of "lost threads" of IUDs

Pregnant	Not pregnant
Unrecognized expulsion + pregnancy	Unrecognized expulsion + not yet pregnant
Perforation + pregnancy	Perforation + not yet pregnant
Device in situ + pregnancy	Device in situ + malpositioned or threads short (in uterus, if not found in cervical canal)

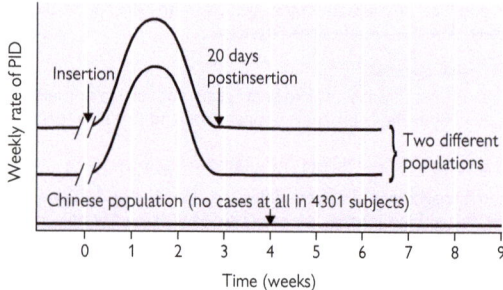

Figure 26.2 WHO study in 1992 of 22,908 IUD insertions (4301 in China) in Europe, Africa, Asia, and the Americas. Note that the weekly rate of pelvic inflammatory disease (PID) returns to preinsertion background rate for the population studied. *Source:* Guillebaud J (2004). *Contraception Today.* New York: Martin Dunitz, p. 27.

Clinical implications for IUD insertion arrangements
- Prospective IUD users should be verbally screened, i.e., a good sexual history needs to be taken (Chapter 1, 📖 p. 8). They need to know that they will, at least, need to use condoms if there is an STD risk.
- If the woman has had sex with more than one male partner in the last 3 months, then the IUD may not be the appropriate contraception.
- A question that needs to be asked but is often left out of the sexual history is, "Do you ever wonder if your partner has or is likely to have another sexual relationship?"
- In populations with a high prevalence of *Chlamydia trachomatis*, this type of history-taking should be backed up by modern DNA-based (LCR or PCR) prescreening. This would be as important for reinsertions as for initial IUD insertions.
- Recent exposure history or evidence of a purulent discharge from the cervix indicates referral for more detailed investigation.
- If *Chlamydia* is detected, the woman should
- Be investigated for linked pathogens,
- Be given necessary treatment and have contact tracing arranged, and
- Have the IUD insertion postponed.

In emergency contraception cases
Screen but treat anyway before the result is available (e.g., with azithromycin 1 g stat).

The cervix should be cleansed very thoroughly (primarily physically, by swabbing) before any device is inserted, with minimum trauma, following the manufacturer's instructions.

In addition to the routine 6-week follow-up visit, a first postinsertion visit might be appropriate at 1–2 weeks, designed to identify any postinsertion infection (during the crucial 20 days of Fig. 26.2).

At a minimum, the woman should be given clear details of the relevant symptoms of PID and instructed to contact her health care provider ~1 week postinsertion.

Actinomyces-like organisms (ALOs)

These are sometimes reported in cervical smears, more commonly with increasing duration of use of either an IUD or IUS. If reported, follow the *relevant* protocols under A, B, and C.

A
- First, call the woman in for an extra consultation and examination; the exam should be done bimanually. If all is normal, see section below on no positive clinical findings, but:
- If there are relevant symptoms or signs (pain, dyspareunia, excessive discharge, tenderness, any suggestion of an adnexal mass), an ultrasound scan should then be arranged, with a low threshold for gynecological referral.
- After preliminary discussion with the microbiologist, the device should be removed and sent for culture. Treatment will have to be vigorous, usually prolonged, if frank pelvic actinomycosis is actually confirmed. It is a potentially life-threatening and fertility-destroying condition, although very rare.

B
When there are no positive clinical findings, in consultation with the woman, the clinician may decide between EITHER
- Simple removal, with or without reinsertion, and without antibiotic treatment
- Advising the woman, along with written reference material, about the relevant symptoms that should make her seek a doctor urgently and tell them that she recently had an IUD or IUS plus ALOs
- Repeating a cervical smear after 3 months (it will nearly always be negative) with a recheck bimanual examination. Both smear-taking and IUD follow-up then revert to normal arrangements.

OR

C
- Leaving the IUD or IUS alone after the initial thorough and fully reassuring examination, preferably backed by a negative pelvic ultrasound scan
- Advising the woman, along with written material, about the relevant symptoms that should make her seek a doctor urgently and tell them that she has been followed up for an IUD or IUS plus ALOs
- Arranging meticulous follow-up, initially at 6 months, including a check for symptoms and bimanual examination

🖙 Given the data that device removal usually clears the ALO finding, even though long-term use is normally best, there is much to be said for following plan A+B rather than A+C.

In either case, keep a good-quality record of the consultation.

Is ectopic pregnancy caused by copper IUDs?

Ectopic pregnancies are actually reduced in number in women with IUDs because very few sperm get through the copper-containing uterine fluids to reach an egg, so very few implantations can occur in any damaged tube. However, there are even fewer implantations in the uterus. Thus, in the ratio of ectopic-to-intrauterine pregnancies, the denominator is even lower than the numerator, allowing the ratio to increase, even though both types of pregnancy are actually reduced in frequency.

A past history is a WHO 3 relative contraindication to the IUD in a nulliparous woman, since there are even better options that are anovulants, e.g., COC, Cerazette®, and DMPA.

The LNG-IUS is also relatively contraindicated, though only WHO 2. See p. 175.

Any IUD user with pain and a late or unusually light period or irregular bleeding has an ectopic pregnancy until proved otherwise.

Pain and bleeding

Copper devices increase
- The *duration* of bleeding by a mean of 1–2 days, and
- The measured *volume* of bleeding by about one-third.

However, if her periods are initially light and of short duration, any addition may be hardly noticeable by the woman.

Bleeding problems usually settle with time. If they do not, it may be necessary to change the method of contraception, perhaps to the LNG-IUS (see next section).

Duration of use

Any copper device (even a copper wire–only type) that has been fitted above the age of 40 may be used for the rest of reproductive life. It never needs replacement, even though it is not licensed for that long. For duration of use of the LNG-IUS in various situations, see the next section.

Cancer risk?

There is no increased cancer risk with IUD use.

The levonorgestrel-releasing intrauterine system (LNG-IUS, or Mirena®)

This LNG-IUS Mirena® is produced by Schering Health Care. The LNG-IUS is shown in Fig. 26.3.

Method of action and effectiveness
The main features of the LNG-IUS are presented in Box 26.2.

Advantages and indications
The user of this method can expect the following advantages:
- A dramatic reduction in the amount and, after the first few months (discussed later), duration of blood loss
- Dysmenorrhea is improved in most women as are (for unexplained reasons) the symptoms of premenstrual syndrome (PMS) in some.
- The LNG-IUS is the contraceptive method of choice for most women with menorrhagia or who are prone to iron-deficiency anemia. Even when there is no need for contraception, it should still be seen in primary care as the first-line treatment for excessively heavy menses without major cavity distortion, and is fully licensed as such.
- *HRT:* by providing progestogenic protection of the uterus during estrogen replacement by any chosen route, it uniquely, before final ovarian failure, offers a "forgettable" contraceptive, no period, and no PMS-type HRT. For this increasingly popular indication, the LNG-IUS is currently licensed for 4 years before it must be replaced.
- *Epilepsy:* in a small series at the MPC, this was a very successful method for treating epilepsy, even in women on enzyme inducer treatment.

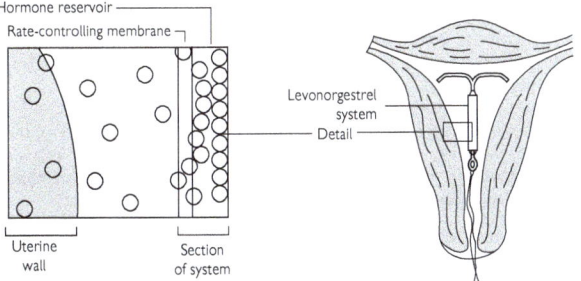

Figure 26.3 The levonorgestrel-releasing intrauterine system (LNG-IUS). Reproduced from *The Pill*, part of the Facts series. 6th edition. By permission of Oxford University Press.

Box 26.2 Main features of the LNG-IUS

- It releases ~20 mcg per 24 hours of LNG from its polydimethylsiloxane reservoir, through a rate-limiting membrane, for its licensed 5 years (and longer).
- Its main contraceptive effects are local, through changes to the cervical mucus and uterotubal fluid, which impair sperm migration, backed by endometrial changes impeding implantation.
- Its cumulative failure rate at 7 years was very low: 1.1 per 100 women in the large Sivin study, and even less at 5 years in the 1994 European multicenter trial.
- Its efficacy is not detectably impaired by enzyme-inducing drugs.
- The systemic blood levels of LNG are under half the mean levels in users of the LNG POP (for users this can be explained as like taking three old-type POPs per week). Although ovarian function is altered in some women, especially in the first year, 85% show the ultrasound changes of normal ovulation at 1 year.
- The amount of LNG in the blood is still enough to give unwanted hormone-type side effects in some women; otherwise irregular light bleeding is the main problem.
- Even if they become amenorrheic, as many do, primarily through a local end-organ effect, in those who do not ovulate (as well as the majority who do), sufficient estrogen is produced for bone health.
- Return of fertility after removal is rapid and appears to be complete.

The LNG-IUS is, in short, a highly convenient and "forgettable" contraceptive, with added gynecological value.

Risk of infection or ectopic pregnancy, risk to future fertility

- LNG-IUS may actually reduce the frequency of clinical PID, perhaps through the progestogenic effect on cervical mucus, particularly in the youngest age groups who are most at risk.
- However, the risk is not eliminated and (outside of mutual monogamy) condom use should still be advocated.
- Future fertility is most unlikely to be adversely affected.
- *Reduction in ectopic risk* can be attributed to the greater efficacy of the sperm-blocking mechanism that reduces the risk of pregnancy in any site. However, ectopics still rarely occur, and with a past history of an ectopic pregnancy, an anovulant method would be even better.

Problems and disadvantages of the LNG-IUS

As with any IUD, *expulsion* can occur and there is the usual small risk of *perforation*. This is minimized by its "withdrawal" as opposed to "plunger" technique of insertion.

A more important problem is the high incidence of *uterine bleeding* in the first postinsertion months. Although small in quantity, it may be very frequent or continuous and can cause considerable inconvenience.

In later months, *amenorrhea* is common but should be explained as being an advantage.

Women can accept the early weeks of light bleeding, even if very frequent, as a worthwhile price to pay for all of the other advantages of the method, provided they are well informed in advance of LNG-IUS fitting.

Women should also be forewarned that although this method is mainly local in its action, it is not exclusively so. Therefore, there is a small incidence of "hormonal" side effects, such as bloating, acne, and depression. These usually improve, often within 2 months, in parallel with the known decline in the higher initial LNG blood levels.

Functional ovarian cysts are also more common, although they are usually asymptomatic. If pain results, they should be investigated and monitored but will usually resolve spontaneously.

Contraindications

Many of the contraindications of this method are the same as those for copper IUDs (see Box 26.1). The additional few that are unique to LNG-IUS, given the actions of its LNG hormone, are listed in Box 26.3.

In addition, the LNG-IUS should not be used as a postcoital intrauterine contraceptive (failures reported). Using a hormone, it appears not to act as quickly as the intrauterine copper ion does.

Relative contraindications for copper IUDs also apply to the LNG-IUS method, but are usually less strong, except for bleeding and pain, which are positive indications (WHO 1).

Duration of use of the LNG-IUS in older women

The product is licensed for 5 years.

For *contraception*, effective use is evidence based but not approved for up to 7 years. For a woman under age 35, because of her greater fertility, replacement after the usual 5 years would be advisable. If fitted above that age, it might be used for longer, even to 7 years after informed consent.

A woman above the age of 45 with complete amenorrhea may continue to use the same LNG-IUS until contraception is no longer needed.

As *part of HRT*, current practice for safe endometrial protection would be always to change it at 4 years.

But if the LNG-IUS is not being and will not be used for either contraception or HRT, it could be left in situ for as long as it continues to work in the control of heavy and/or painful uterine bleeding and then removed after ovarian failure can be finally assured.

Box 26.3 Unique contraindications for LNG-IUS

- Current liver tumor or severe active hepatocellular disease
- Current severe active arterial disease
- ♦* Breast cancer
- Trophoblastic disease (any)—contraindicated while blood hCG levels are high, as for other progestogen-only methods, but there is no problem after full recovery
- Hypersensitivity to levonorgestrel or other constituent

Main established contraindications to IUDs
These apply to the LNG-IUS as well, except where stated.

Absolute, but perhaps temporary, contraindications (WHO 4) for IUD
- Suspicion of pregnancy
- Undiagnosed irregular genital tract bleeding
- Significant infection: postseptic abortion, current pelvic infection or STD, undiagnosed pelvic tenderness or deep dyspareunia, or purulent cervical discharge
- Significant immunosuppression, i.e., more profound than merely use of low-dose corticosteroids
- Malignant or benign trophoblastic disease, while hCG abnormal
- Breast cancer; this might be an indication for copper IUD

Absolute permanent contraindications (WHO 4) for IUDs
- Markedly distorted uterine cavity or cavity sounding to <5 cm depth
- Known true allergy to a constituent
- Wilson's disease (copper IUDs only)
- Pulmonary hypertension, because of risk of fatal vasovagal reaction through cervical instrumentation
- Previous endocarditis or after prosthetic valve replacement (LNG-IUS can be WHO 3 for these, as it is believed the progestogen effect on mucus reduces the risk of infection or endocarditis. But full antibiotic cover is required for insertion, see point 8 below).

Relative contraindications (WHO 2 unless otherwise stated) for IUDs
These constitute a longish list, but in general, an IUD or the LNG-IUS is usable with caution. Note again the differences specific to the LNG-IUS.

1. *Nulliparity and young age*, especially <20 years. This contraindication is due to of the risk of infection and its more serious implications, should that happen. Both the IUD and the IUS are used successfully by many (carefully selected) women.
2. Lifestyle of self or partner(s) *risking STDs*
3. Past *history of definite pelvic infection*
4. Recent *exposure to high risk of a STD*
    - In emergency situations, such as for postcoital contraception, a copper IUD may be permissible with full antibiotic cover (and after microbiological swabs have been taken).
5. Known *HIV infection*. While controlled by drug therapy HIV is only a relative contraindication, depending on the risk of contracting a new STD. The LNG-IUS is a better choice because of reduced blood loss (added condom use is routinely advised).
6. *Past history of ectopic pregnancy* or other history suggesting a high ectopic risk in a nulliparous woman. T-Safe Cu 380A® or LNG-IUS are preferred IUDs, but regardless of parity, it is even better to use an anovulant contraceptive.
7. *Suspected subfertility* already

8. *Structural heart disease with risk of endocarditis* but no history thereof (see above), signifying the need for full antibiotic cover for IUD or IUS insertion. The LNG-IUS is probably better for these cases than a copper IUD, as it is believed to pose less ongoing infection risk because of the mucus effect.
9. *Any prosthesis* that can be prejudiced by blood-borne infection, e.g., hip replacement. IUDs are usable, but with antibiotic coverage for the insertion.
10. *Postpartum*, between 48 hours and 4 weeks (excess risk of perforation)
11. *Fibroids or congenital abnormality of the uterus* with some but not marked distortion of the uterine cavity (see p. 140)
12. Severely *scarred or distorted uterus*, e.g., after myomectomy
13. After *endometrial ablation or resection*. There is a risk of the IUD becoming stuck in a shrunken and scarred cavity. The LNG-IUS is usable in selected cases.
14. *Heavy periods*, with or without anemia before insertion for any reason, including anticoagulation. This is an indication for the LNG-IUS.
15. *Dysmenorrhea*, any type. LNG-IUS may well benefit this candidate.
16. *Endometriosis* may be benefited by LNG-IUS, to help alleviate local symptoms in addition to providing systemic treatment.
17. *Diabetes*. Three is a small risk of infection, but the IUD and LNG-IUS can be excellent choices.
18. *Previous perforation of uterus* is low risk, at least for the small defect in the uterine fundus after a previous IUD perforation. Healing is so complete, usually within 3 months, that it is difficult to locate the site of the previous event.
19. (LNG-IUS only) *Liver tumor or cancer* (rare but possible because there is some systemic progestogen)

Counseling, insertion, and follow-up

Timing of insertions—all intrauterine contraceptives

Generally, *in the normal cycle*, timing must avoid an already implanted pregnancy. With copper IUDs (because they are such efficient postcoital methods), insertion can be at any time up to 5 days after the calculated day of ovulation, but not so with the LNG-IUS (see below).

Postpartum insertions of IUDs or IUSs are usually at 6 weeks and acceptable from 4 weeks (beware of increased risk of perforation). After 4 weeks, if the woman is not fully breastfeeding, conception risk should be discussed (p. 178) and additional contraception advised for 7 days.

- Following first-trimester abortion (but only after preliminary counseling and full agreement by the woman), immediate insertion is best on the day of surgically induced abortion or second part of a medical abortion, if the uterus is clearly empty. This can be checked by on-the-spot ultrasound.

Additional points about insertion timing for the LNG-IUS

Insertion for the IUS should be no later than day 7 of the normal cycle, since it does not operate as an effective postcoital contraceptive and because any fetus might be harmed by conception in the first cycle (there is a very high local LNG concentration).

Later insertion is also acceptable, but only if there has been believable abstinence beforehand and with continued contraception (e.g., condoms) postinsertion for 7 days.

If a woman is on the COC or POP or DMPA, the IUS can normally be inserted at any time, with no added precautions. As with Implanon® (p. 243), it is ideal to arrange that one of those methods is in use at the time of IUS-fitting.

Counseling and follow-up (for both IUDs and IUS)

After considering the contraindications, there should be an unhurried discussion with the woman of all the main practical points about this method. The focus should be on infection risk and the importance of reporting pain as a symptom at any time and of contacting her physician if it occurs in the first 3 weeks postinsertion.

The only important routine follow-up visit is usually at 6 weeks after insertion. This is to

- Discuss with the woman any menstrual (or other) symptoms;
- Check for (partial) expulsion;
- Exclude infection, i.e., no relevant symptoms, tenderness or mass.

According to the WHO, there is no need for planned visits thereafter, until the next scheduled annual exam. This is fine for copper IUDs, but extra visits in early months can sometimes be helpful for LNG-IUS users to maintain their motivation until any breakthrough bleeding resolves.

Training for the actual insertion process

Good analgesia is crucial:

- Premedication with a nonsteroidal, e.g., Motrin 600, prior to insertion should be routine for all insertions.
- Local anesthesia by intracervical injection should be taught and offered as a choice. It should almost always be used if the cervix has to be dilated or the uterine cavity explored.
- Moreover, any woman (even a relaxed parous woman) may experience a very unpredictable but sometimes bad pain that is caused by application of the tenaculum at 12 o'clock on the cervix. An initial 1 mL dose of 1% lidocaine completely abolishes this.

Chapter 27

Postcoital contraception

Introduction *262*
Levonorgestrel emergency contraception (LNG-EC) *263*
Copper intrauterine devices (IUDs) *264*
Counseling and management *265*
Special indications for EC *267*

CHAPTER 27 Postcoital contraception

Introduction

Three methods have now been shown to be effective contraceptives when initiated *after* unprotected sexual intercourse (UPSI):
- Insertion of a copper intrauterine device (IUD)
- Combined oral emergency contraceptive (COEC) using levonorgestrel (LNG) 500 mcg + ethinylestradiol (EE) 100 mcg repeated in 12 hours
- Levonorgestrel progestogen-only emergency contraceptive (here shortened to LNG-EC) given as a stat dose of LNG 1500 mcg. See Table 27.1.

Table 27.1 Emergency contraception: choice of methods

	LNG-EC	Copper IUD
	LNG 1.5 mg as stat dose	Immediate insertion, but sometimes better to delay (see text)
Normal timing after intercourse	Up to 72 hours but also usable up to 120 hours (see text)	Up to 5 days, or 5 days after earliest calculated day of ovulation
Efficacy (overall) within 72 hours	~99%	About 99.9%
Side effects	Nausea 23% (15%) Vomiting 6% (1.4%)	Pain, bleeding, risk of infection

Reprinted with permission from Elsevier. Task Force on Postovulatory Methods of Fertility Regulation. Randomised controlled trial of levonorgestrel versus the Yuzpe regimen of combined oral contraceptives for emergency contraception. *The Lancet* 1998; 352:428–433, and WHO. *The Lancet* 2002; 360:1803–1810. (This study showed the lower rate of side effects in parentheses.)

Levonorgestrel emergency contraception (LNG-EC)

Mechanism of action
- *Given at or before ovulation,* the method interferes with follicle development, either inhibiting altogether or delaying ovulation.
- *Given later in a cycle* it is capable of inhibiting implantation, but this seems to be the less effective of its mechanisms, so the failure rate tends to be higher for sexual exposures late in the cycle.

Effectiveness and advantages
- Greater effectiveness: 99.6% when treatment began *within 24 hours of a single exposure,* compared with 98% for COEC
- Reduced rates of the main side effects of nausea and vomiting
- In ordinary practice, there are virtually no contraindications to it.

The apparent effectiveness of LNG-EC with treatment up to 72 hours after a single sexual exposure is ~99%, but this represents prevention of only 80% of the expected pregnancies, since most of those who present would not actually have conceived.

Enzyme inducer drug (EID) treatment
If the woman is taking an EID, it would be better to use an alternative, in this case:
- Insertion of a copper IUD (the more effective option), or if that is not acceptable,
- The dose should be doubled, i.e., two tablets totalling 3 mg stat (unlicensed use).

Warfarin users should have their INR checked 3–4 days after LNG-EC, since it may alter significantly.

Contraindications
Very few absolute medical contraindications to the hormone methods exist, except:
- Current pregnancy
- Proven severe allergy or intolerance to a constituent
- Active acute porphyria, with a past attack precipitated by sex hormones
- If the woman's own ethics preclude intervention postcoitally (or, more relevantly, postimplantation, see p. 257).

Relative contraindications
- EID treatment, see earlier discussion.
- Current breast cancer (but adverse effect is unlikely with such short exposure)
- Trophoblastic disease with high hCG levels (adverse effect is unlikely given the immediate risks of pregnancy)
- In breastfeeding, conception risk is usually very low, so EC treatment would rarely be needed. If it is indicated, the infant could be bottle-fed for 24 hours, with expression of the breast milk.

Copper intrauterine devices (IUDs)

Insertion of a copper IUD—not the LNG-IUS—before implantation is extremely effective, through the toxicity of copper ions to sperm or by blocking implantation. This means, after consultation with the woman, that insertion may proceed, up to 5 days after
- The first sexual exposure (regardless of cycle length) or
- The (earliest) calculated ovulation day. This entails the following:
  - Calculate the *soonest likely* next menstrual start day;
  - Subtract 14 days for mean life of the corpus luteum; and
  - Add 5 days to allow for mean interval from fertilization to implantation.

Effectiveness
The copper IUD prevents conception in ~99.9% of women who present, or 98% of those who might be expected otherwise to conceive—even in cases of multiple exposure since the last menstrual period.

Indications for EC by copper IUD
In selected individuals (see Box 27.1) IUD insertion may be ideal.

Clinically, given the sexual history, insertion in most cases should occur
- After microbiological cervical screening (at least for *Chlamydia trachomatis*) and
- With prophylactic antibiotic cover, e.g., with azithromycin 1 g stat, and
- With close follow-up if sexually transmitted disease (STD) test results later prove positive.

Box 27.1 Ideal use of copper IUD
- When maximum efficacy is the woman's priority.
- When exposure occurred >72 hours earlier, or in cases of multiple exposure: insertion may occur
  - Up to 5 days after the earliest UPSI at any time in a cycle or
  - If there have been many UPSI acts, no later than 5 days after calculated ovulation.
- To be retained as long-term method of contraception
- When there are contraindications to the hormonal method
- If the woman is currently vomiting, or if she unexpectedly vomits her dose of LNG-EC within 2 hours, in a case with a particularly high pregnancy risk

Counseling and management

- Preserve confidentiality.
- Evaluate the possibility of sexual assault or rape.
- Using a good leaflet as the basis for discussion, help the woman to make a fully informed and autonomous choice.

The decision could be *either* of the two EC methods *or* taking no action postcoitally.

Pharmacists should ensure privacy for the discussion and have a low threshold for referring all cases outside their specified purview (e.g., >72 hours since the earliest UPSI), to an appropriate health care provider.

Careful assessment of *menstrual and coital history* is essential.

Contraindications

The mode of action may itself pose the only contraindication or problem for some individuals.

Sometimes it may help to explain that there are circumstances when LNG-EC's powerful prefertilization effects can remove concern about it needing to use the postfertilization mechanism (e.g., if the treatment is clearly going to be given well before ovulation in a given cycle—even though postcoitus).

Medical risks

These should be discussed, especially the following:
- *Failure rate* (see p. 267), reminding the woman that these figures relate to a single exposure. The failure rate is very close to nil for the IUD method.
- *Teratogenicity* is believed to be negligible.
- *Ectopic pregnancy*. If this occurs, the EC was not causative.

However:
- A past history of ectopic pregnancy or pelvic infection remains a reason for specific forewarning with any of the methods.
- All women should be warned to report back urgently if they experience pain. Providers must think "ectopic" whenever LNG-EC or a copper IUD fails or there is an odd bleeding pattern post-treatment.

Side effects
Nausea occurs in 15%, vomiting in 1.4% of users. If the contraceptive dose is vomited within 2 hours, the woman may be given a further tablet with an antiemetic.

Contraception

Contraception, in both the current cycle (in case the LNG-EC method merely postpones ovulation), which often involves condoms, and long term, should be discussed. The IUD option may cover both aspects (for a suitable long-term user).

If the COC or injectable is chosen, it should be started as soon as the woman is convinced her next period is normal, usually on the first or second day, without the need for additional contraception thereafter.

But "quick start" of the COC is also an option in selected cases. This means starting a COC immediately after the EC, along with advice for 7 days of added condom use and 100% follow-up.

The clinician must be confident that the benefits (especially to future compliance) outweigh the risks of EC failure.

Follow-up

Women receiving LNG-EC should be instructed to return
- If they experience pain or
- If their expected period is >7 days late or lighter than usual.

IUD users return usually in 4–6 weeks for a routine checkup, or perhaps for device removal, in order for them to establish a more appropriate long-term method.

Special indications for EC

These apply to coital exposure when the following have occurred:
- Omission of anything more than two COC tablets after the pill-free interval, or of more than two pills in the first seven in the packet.
- Delay in taking a POP tablet for >3 hours, outside of lactation, implying loss of the mucus effect, followed by sexual exposure before contraception was restored. The POP is restarted immediately after the emergency regimen; 2 days of added precautions are advised; and follow-up is agreed on.
- If the POP user is breastfeeding, EC would only be indicated if either the breastfeeding or the POP-taking were unusually inadequate (p. 224).
- Removal or expulsion of an IUD before the time of implantation, if another IUD cannot be inserted for some reason
- Further exposure in the same cycle, e.g., due to failure of barrier contraception >1 day after a dose of EC has been taken. Additional courses of LNG-EC may be clinically indicated, given reasonable precautions to avoid treating after implantation (repeated use thereafter will not induce an abortion).

This use is again outside the terms of the licence.

Use of LNG-EC later than 72 hours after earliest UPSI
This possibility has been tested in an RCT by the WHO (2002; p. 263). The failure rate was low: only eight failures in 314 women treated between 72 and 120 hours (5 days) after the earliest act of UPSI. Although this was a small study and the confidence intervals were wide, it provides sufficient evidence for LNG-EC to be offered to selected women in the 72- to 120-hour time period.

They should be told of the limited evidence of efficacy, though it is likely to be better than doing nothing. They should also be informed that a copper IUD would definitely be more effective.

Overdue injections of DMPA with continuing sexual intercourse
If it is later than day 91 (end of the 13th week), after a negative sensitive pregnancy test, LNG-EC may be given along with the next injection plus advice to use condoms for 7 days.

But after day 98 (14 weeks), the next injection is best postponed until there has been a total of 14 days of safe contraception or abstinence since the last sexual exposure and a sensitive (<25 mIU/L) pregnancy test is negative—again, with 7 days' added precautions and good follow-up.

In all circumstances of use of EC, the women should be aware that
- The method might fail.
- It is not an abortifacient.
- It is given too soon to be able to harm a baby.

Chapter 28

Sterilization

Introduction 270
Efficacy considerations 271
Potential reversibility 272
Possible long-term side effects of female sterilization 273
Comparison of methods 274

Introduction

Many individuals who say it is impossible to continue use of reversible contraceptives may just need an update on other methods of contraception in order to correct misinformation about the greater effectiveness and added advantages of current options (above all, the LNG-IUS, but also the T-Safe 380 A® IUD and Implanon®).

Deferment or even avoidance of surgery is often ideal, through careful discussion and explanation of alternatives, particularly the long-acting reversible methods (LARCs).

Efficacy considerations

Sterilization

The overall failure rate is ~0.2–0.3%, or a lifetime risk of 3 failures per 1000 procedures. A follow-up study of 10,685 women in the United States over 8–14 years who used a variety of sterilization methods established that the failure rate of tubal sterilization, however performed, does not stabilize after 2 years.

The increased risk that any failure that occurred might be ectopic should be specifically explained. For vasectomy, a much lower late-failure rate can be quoted, namely 1 case in 2000, after negative semen testing at least 3 months after surgery.

Cauterization is effective and easily preformed but has a low incidence of reversal.

Other types of tubal occlusion include the following:
- Falope rings and Filshie clip—a small silastic band or clip is placed around a loop of fallopian tube. This method has a higher complication rate and failure rate than that of a Filshie clip.
- Pomeroy technique—this involves the removal of a portion of the fallopian tube. Again, there is a higher incidence of interoperative and postoperative bleeding, and it is more difficult to reverse.

Essure

This is a permanent transcervical sterilization procedure developed by Conceptus, Inc., that is 99.74% effective and is more cost-effective than a bilateral tubal ligation. Microinserts are placed in the fallopian tube via a catheter and contain polyethylene terephthalate that elicit scarring over a period of 3 months. Ultimately, an occlusion is formed blocking sperm.

A second form of birth control must be used after the procedure for 3 months until the effectiveness can be confirmed.

Vasectomy

Vasectomy is a safe, easy, effective, permanent, and affordable alternative to bilateral tubal ligation. The vas deferens are cut and then sutured, preventing sperm from leaving the epididymis.

The procedure takes about 30 minutes and is often performed in the physician's office.
- One out of five men in the United States over the age of 35 has undergone a vasectomy.
- It is successful in more than 99% of men.
- The patient must ejaculate 20 times after the procedure to clear the ducts, and then the ejaculate is tested 8 weeks after surgery
- Complications are unusual but can include bleeding, infection, sperm granuloma, sperm congestion, and/or formation of sperm antibodies.
- Vasovasostomy (vasectomy reversal) is the reconnection of the vas deferens and is successful 76% of the time if performed within 3 years of the vasectomy. An alternative option is sperm banking prior to vasectomy.

Potential reversibility

Reported success of *reversal* procedures (male or female) depends enormously on patient selection, especially:
- How much damage was done at the initial procedure
- The age of the woman in the new relationship
- For vasectomy, time elapsed since surgery (poor results beyond 10 years)

With competent microsurgery, as a rule of thumb, 80–90% of tubal patency is usual.[1] This surgery is not available everywhere and is usually expensive. It is wise, therefore, to proceed with sterilization only when both partners can fully accept its permanence.

---

1 Winston RM (1977). Microsurgical tubocornual anastomosis for reversal of sterilisation. *Lancet* 1:284–285.

Possible long-term side effects of female sterilization

The psychological sequelae
Considerable regret has been reported in 2% of patients at 6 months and by 4% at 18 months, and postoperative psychiatric disturbance and dissatisfaction were largely associated with preoperative psychiatric disturbance.

Higher rates of regret are reported when sterilization is done at times that are not, except in rare special cases, now recommended: at termination of pregnancy or Caesarean section, or immediately postpartum.

Menstrual irregularity or menorrhagia
Sterilization, male or female, does not affect menstrual loss. However, if the method of contraception prior to the sterilization was COC, then the lighter regular withdrawal bleeds of the COC are replaced by normal menstruation.

Therefore, counseling MUST include specific questioning about whether heavy bleeding or pain are or were problems during the woman's natural cycles, even if this relates to many years ago. Only with this information can the right decision be made, which could be to use the LNG-IUS instead of either party undergoing sterilization.

Ovarian cancer
In several studies it appears that tubal sterilization may reduce the risk of ovarian cancer. This possible beneficial side effect is difficult to explain, but may be a real effect.

Likelihood of regret following sterilization
A study in 1980 of women undergoing reversal of sterilization found the following:
- 87% were under the age of 30. In the Unites States, marriages or intended long-term relationships started under age 25 have a failure rate of >50%.
- 63% had been sterilized after delivery
- No less than 75% had been unhappy in their relationship.

It is important that any disharmony with or pressuring by the partner be identified. Easily missed, these factors may more likely be noted by the referring clinician in primary care than by the hospital gynecologist or surgeon.

Comparison of methods

Vasectomy

Vasectomy is a very simple procedure and is medically safe under local anesthesia. The method of choice is "no scalpel vasectomy."

Sperm testing is usually done 12–16 weeks postsurgery, for two reasons:
- To establish clearance of "downstream sperm
- To exclude early failures of the procedure (incidence ~1%)

Clinically, men choosing vasectomy should be specifically advised
- In the short term about occasional large postoperative hematomas
- Longer term, about chronic postvasectomy scrotal pain. A surprisingly high incidence of this has been reported in some studies. Less than 1% of men seek medical help for this or report that it noticeably affects their quality of life. It rarely seems to cause regret about having had the vasectomy.

Despite periodic concerns about a link to testicular or prostate cancer, no long-term systemic risks have been established.

Tubal occlusion

Tubal occlusion remains a more invasive procedure with a risk of intra-abdominal injury even when performed under local anesthesia.

Tubal occlusion confers immediate sterility (provided fertilization has not already occurred that cycle), while it may take several months before the semen is clear of sperm after the male operation.

Chapter 29

Special considerations

How can a provider be reasonably sure of a woman not being pregnant? *276*
Contraception at the climacteric *278*

How can a health care provider be reasonably sure of a woman not being pregnant?

The health care provider can be reasonably certain that the woman is not pregnant if she has no symptoms or signs of pregnancy and one or more of the following criteria apply:
- She has not had intercourse since last normal menses.
- She has been correctly and consistently using a reliable method of contraception.
- She is within the first 7 days after (onset of) normal menses.
- She is within 4 weeks postpartum for nonlactating women.
- She is within the first 7 days postabortion or miscarriage.

These criteria should be backed by a urine pregnancy test with sensitivity of at least 25 IU/L, best done on a concentrated early-morning sample.

Quick start

Quick start is the immediate starting of (usually) a contraceptive pill method at first visit, late in the menstrual cycle. This may often be an entirely appropriate use, but only when the above criteria have been applied, so that the provider can be reasonably sure of a woman not being pregnant nor about to be pregnant.

Secondary amenorrhea, wants to (re)start contraception

This situation is where the greatest difficulty arises, e.g.:
- Not breastfeeding and beyond 4 weeks postpartum, without reliable contraception to date
- A woman >2 weeks overdue for her DMPA injection

Often, a pair of visits may be required, since a prediagnosable pregnancy (unimplanted blastocyst) might be present at the first visit.

First visit

Take a history of early symptoms of pregnancy (increased micturition, nausea) and perform a urine pregnancy test with sensitivity of at least 25 IU/L (only) if the history is suggestive.

If this test is negative and there are no symptoms and IF more assurance is required before taking action (as, for example, before inserting an LNG-IUS):
- Recommend that she abstain from intercourse (preferable) or
- Teach her to use a back-up method such as condoms with exceptional care.
- ☙ If neither of these options is appropriate, given that POPs have never been suspected of harming an early pregnancy, one of these may be prescribed.

She needs to use one of these contraceptive methods UNTIL at least 14 days have elapsed since whenever her last unprotected intercourse occurred.

She should return to the clinic at that time, bringing an early-morning urine sample. But if a pill method is planned, she may be given supplies in case her period starts and she can start the pill regimen at home as usual.

Second visit
- If she returns after menses, start any chosen method (including IUD or IUS) in the usual manner.
- If she returns still amenorrheic, do a pregnancy test.

If now:
- She has no symptoms of pregnancy plus
- Pregnancy test with sensitivity ≤25 IU/L is negative and
- The back-up method has reportedly been used well.

provide the (new) contraceptive method. If it is hormonal, advise usual contraceptive back-up for 7 days, or for 2 days with a POP.

Given that in 10–15% of cases a sensitive pregnancy test 14 days postcoitally can be falsely negative, arrange for a further follow-up in 2–4 weeks to confirm her nonpregnant state. Or at least instruct the woman to return if she develops symptoms that could signal a pregnancy, or if she fails to see her first withdrawal bleed on the COC.

Contraception at the climacteric

Maximum age for COC use

Smokers or others with arterial risk factors

These women should always discontinue the COC at age 35. Pending more data, if they request a hormonal contraceptive, they should use a POP or implant, but an IUD or IUS would be even better, or a vasectomy for their partner.

In selected healthy, migraine-free nonsmokers, with modern pills and careful monitoring, the many gynecological and other benefits of COCs are now felt to outweigh the small, though increasing, cardiovascular (and breast cancer) risk of use of a modern pill up to age 50–51, which is the mean age of menopause.

Although there are usually much better contraceptive choices—consider especially an intrauterine method—an appropriate COC (usually a 20 mcg product) may be used until then. For women with diminishing ovarian function but who still need contraception, this is logical and preferable to HRT, along with use of some other contraceptive (though not advised beyond about age 50, see below).

Beyond 50 years of age

The age-related increased COC risks are usually unacceptable for all women, given that fertility is now so low that simple, virtually risk-free contraceptives will suffice, e.g., spermicides, sponges, or the POP.

Most forms of HRT are not contraceptive but may be indicated combined with a simple contraceptive in symptomatic women when estrogen is no longer being supplied by the COC. The IUS plus HRT combination is a good choice here, since before final ovarian failure it safely supplies contraceptive HRT with endometrial protection plus, usually, highly acceptable amenorrhea.

Diagnosing loss of fertility at menopause

Although hormones, including the POP, tend to mask menopause, it is not always necessary to know the precise time of final ovarian failure. Moreover, FSH levels are unreliable for diagnosis of complete loss of ovarian function. So one of the options in Box 29.1 should be followed.

Box 29.1 Contraception cessation

Contraception may cease: after waiting for 1 year of amenorrhea above age 50, having stopped all hormones

This is the obvious plan for women using the following:
- Copper IUDs
- Condoms
- Sponge or spermicides (which, unlike in younger women, appear to be adequate in the presence of such drastically reduced if not absent fertility)

But if the woman is using one of the other hormonal methods or HRT, which mask menopause, what are the options?

- If on DMPA or COC (or Evra® patch): age 50 is the time to stop these (and maybe switch to a POP). They are needlessly strong contraceptives and the known risks increase with age.
- The POP, or an implant, or the LNG-IUS, or a sponge or spermicide with ongoing HRT: as contraceptives, these add negligible medical risks that increase with age.

Therefore, one of these (usually the POP) may be continued until the latest age of potential fertility has been reached. Then the woman just stops the contraception. When is that? A good estimate is age 55.

Contraception may cease: above age 50 if three other criteria apply
Older users of hormonal contraception may cease using any method *IF*

1. They have passed their 50th birthday AND, after a trial of 2 months' discontinuation using barriers or spermicides, they have
2. Vasomotor symptoms
3. Two separate high FSH levels (>30 U/L) 1 month apart when off all treatment, and
4. Continuing amenorrhea thereafter beyond this trial period.

With due warnings of lack of certainty, these women may cease all contraception earlier than the approved 1 year after age 50. Or, as before, they should use a sponge or spermicide until 1 year of amenorrhea is finally established.

Appendix

Essential Web sites in reproductive health *282*
Further reading and references *282*

Essential Web sites in reproductive health

www.nih.gov
National Institutes of Health
www.ama-assn.org
American Medical Association
www.asrm.org
American Society for Reproductive Medicine
www.acog.org
American College of Obstetricians and Gynecologists
www.the-bms.org
Research-based advice on menopause and hormone replacement therapy

Further reading and references

Guillebaud J (2003). Contraception. In: McPherson A, Waller D, eds. *Women's Health*, 5th ed. Oxford: Oxford University Press (formerly *Women's Problems in General Practice*).

Guillebaud J (2004). *Contraception—Your Questions Answered*. Edinburgh: Churchill-Livingstone.

National Institute for Health and Clinical Excellence. The effective and appropriate use of long-acting reversible contraception. London: RCOG, October 2005. www.nice.org.uk/pdf/CG030fullguideline.pdf

WHO (2004). *Medical Eligibility Criteria for Contraceptive Use* (WHOMEC). Geneva: WHO.

WHO (2005). *Selected Practice Recommendations for Contraceptive Use* (WHOSPR). Geneva: WHO.

See www.who.int/reproductive-health for both of these.

Index

A

Abnormal embryological development, 7–8
Acne, and PCOS, 47
Actinomyces-like organisms (ALOs), and IUDs, 253
Acute myocardial infarction (AMI), and COCs, 199
Addison disease, 18
Adolescent gynecology, 23
Adrenal cortex, steroids of, 18
Adrenal insufficiency, 18
Adrenal steroid synthesis
  cholesterol, hormones from, 19
  regulation of, 18–20
Adrenocorticotropic hormone (ACTH), 18–20
Alcohol and conception, relationship between, 86
Aldosterone, 19
5-alpha-reductase deficiency, 9
Altitude illness, and COCs, 206–7
Amenorrhea, 61
  definition of, 62
  diagnosis of, 68
  etiology of, 63–6
  history-taking and physical examination checklist for, 67
  investigations of, 67–8
  management of, 70
  and POP, 228
American Society for Reproductive Medicine (ASRM), 158, 42
  classification of Müllerian anomalies, 10–12
Androgens, 18
  and hair growth, 53
  ovarian, excessive production of, 44, 45
  -producing tumors, 56
Androstendione, 53, 75, 19
Anovulation, 42, 47–8
  causes of, 38
  diagnosis of, 68
  treatment possibilities for, 107
Antiandrogen medications, for hirsutism, 58

Antibiotics, long-term use of, 213
Antisperm antibodies, 114
  detection of, 116
Aromatase inhibitors, 125
  for endometriosis, 149
Arterial diseases, and COCs, 199, 202–3
  dosage and hormone type, 199
Asherman's syndrome, 140
Assisted reproductive technologies (ART), 147, 158, 153
  children born as result of, 166
Asthenospermia, 95–7
Autoimmune causes, of male infertility, 114
Azoospermia factor regions, 113

B

Basal body temperature (BBT) chart, 98–9
Benign breast disease (BBD), and COCs, 196
Bilateral vasectomy, 185
Biochemical analysis of seminal fluid, 116
Biosynthesis reactions, of steroid hormones, 18–20
  disorders resulting from defects in, 20
Birth control. See Contraception
Bleeding, and IUDs, 254
Blood pressure monitoring, and COCs, 221
Body mass index (BMI), 98–9
Body weight and conception, relationship between, 86
Bone density, and injectables, 235–7
Bone mass
  factors affecting bone mass, 77
  and menopause, 77–8
Breakthrough bleeding (BTB), 210–11, 216–17
Breast cancer, and COCs, 196

Broad-spectrum antibiotics, and POP, 225
Bromocriptine, for hyperprolactinemia, 70

C

Cabergoline, for hyperprolactinemia, 70
Cancer risk, and IUDs, 254
Caps, 188
  advantages, 189
  disadvantages, 189
  fitting and follow-up, 189
Carbamazepine, 225
Cardiovascular disease, and COCs, 199–204
  prescribing guidelines, 199–204
Cardiovascular risk, and menopause, 78
Central nervous system (CNS), and menopause, 77
Cervical cancer, and COCs, 196–7
Cholesterol, 16
Choriocarcinoma, and COCs, 197
Chromosome analysis, 96
Ciclosporin, 213–14
Circulatory disease, and COCs, 205
Climacteric period, 7.3
  contraception at, 278
  diagnosing loss of fertility at menopause, 278
  maximum age for COC use, 278
Clomifene citrate (CC), 123–4
  adjuvants for, 124
  for anovulation, 47–8
  dose, 123
  duration of treatment, 124
  indications, 123
  mode of action, 123
  monitoring, 124
  side effects of, 124
  results, 123
    factors affecting, 123
  for unexplained infertility, 108
"Clomifene failure," 123
Clonazepam, 213–14

INDEX

Clonidine, 82
Coitus interruptus, 182
  advantages, 182
  disadvantages, 182
  effectiveness, 182
Colorectal cancer, and COCs, 197–8
Combined oral contraceptives (COCs), 170, 193, 214–15
  benefits and risks, 195
  cardiovascular disease and, 199–204
  congenital abnormalities and fertility issues, 222
  counselling and ongoing supervision, 216–19
  discontinuation of, 220
    early, reasons for, 220
    symptoms for, 220
  drug interactions, 212
  for hirsutism, 58
  maximum age for use, 278
  mechanism of action, 194
  pill follow-up, 221
  tumor risk and, 196–8
  WHO eligibility criteria for, 205–11
Complete androgen insensitivity syndrome (CAIS), 9
Conception
  delays in, 83
    environmental and dietary influences, 86
    female partner, age of, 85
  fertility problems, prevalence of, 84
  initial investigation, timing of, 84
  intercourse, frequency and timing of, 85
  rate, 88
Condoms, 178
  male, 183
    advantages and indications, 183
    effectiveness, 183
    problems and disadvantages, 183
  female, 188
Congenital abnormalities, and COCs, 222
Congenital adrenal hyperplasia (CAH), 57, 9
Constitutional delay of growth and puberty, 29
Contraception
  cessation, 279
  male, 181
  postcoital, 261

Contraception patch (Ortho Evra), 221
Contraceptive implants, 239
  advantages, 243
  body mass, effect of, 241
  counselling and ongoing supervision, 245
  bleeding problems, 245
  bone mineral density, 245
  clinical management, 245
  minor side effects, 245
  weight gain, 245
  disadvantages and contraindications, 244
  enzyme inducers treatment, 242
  indications, 243
  mechanism of action, administration and effectiveness, 241
  reversibility and removal problems, 242
Contraceptives
  available methods, effectiveness of, 173, 174
  eligibility criteria for, 175
  ideal, features of, 171, 172
  WHO classification of contraindications, 175, 172
Contraceptive sponges, 178, 190
Contraceptive steroids
  blood levels of, variations in, 217
Contract tracing, 171
Copper intrauterine devices, 170, 178, 249–54, 264
  advantages and indications, 249
  banded IUDs, advantages, 249
  duration of use, 254
  ectopic pregnancy and, 254
  effectiveness, 264
  ideal use of, 264
  indications for EC by, 264
  influence of age on effectiveness, 249
  in situ conception, 250–1
  mechanism of action, 249
  pain and bleeding due to, 254
  problems and disadvantages, 249–50
Coronary heart disease (CHD), and menopause, 78
Corticosterone, 19

Cortisol, 19
  production control, feedback loop for, 19
Counseling, for COCs, 216–19
  new pill taker, take-home messages for, 216
  pill brand, second choice for, 216–17, 217–19
  abnormal bleeding, checklist for, 218
  bleeding side effects, 216–17
  relative estrogen excess, 218
  relative progestogen excess, 218
  starting COCs, 216
Cushing's syndrome, 57
Cystic ovarian endometriosis, 145

D

Danazol, for endometriosis, 149
DAX1 gene, 6
Deep rectosigmoidal endometriosis, 145, 146
Deep rectovaginal endometriosis, 145, 146
Delayed onset of puberty, 29
  causes of, 29
  investigations of, 29
Depot medroxyprogesterone acetate (DMPA), 170, 178, 232, 232
  absolute contraindications for, 237
  cautions in use of, 236
  duration of use, 236–7
  overdue injections, with continuing sexual intercourse, 233–4, 267
  relative contraindications for, 237
  timing of the first injection of, 233
  use for women, 236
Desmolase, 18–20
Dexamethasone, 124
  for LOCAH, 58
Diabetes mellitus (DM), and COCs, 207–8
Diaphragms, 188
  advantages, 189
  disadvantages, 189
  fitting and follow-up, 189
Dihydrotestosterone (DHT), 21

DMRT1 gene, 6
Dopamine agonists, for hyperprolactinemia, 71
Drospirenone, 213–14
Drug interactions
 of COCs, 212
 and POP, 225
Drugs, and male infertility, 114, 115

E

Ectopic pregnancy, and IUDs, 254
"Egg-sharing," 163
Embryo freezing, 162
Embryo transfer (ET), 108, 156, 158, 162
Emergency contraception
 choice of methods, 262
 special indications for, 267
Endocrine causes, of male infertility, 114
Endometriomas, removal versus ablation of, 145
Endometriosis, 141
 -associated infertility, 144
 examination and investigations, 143
 medical treatment for, 148
 side effects of drugs, 150
 surgery principles for infertility patients with, 147
 surgical treatment of, 145–6
Endometrium
 carcinomas of, and COCs, 197
Environmental factors, of male infertility, 114
Enzyme inducer drugs (EID), 212, 263
 and contraceptive implants, 242
 long-term use of, 213–14
 recommended regimen, 214
 and POP, 225
Essure, 271
Estradiol, 16, 21, 34–5
Estrogen, 235, 77, 78, 81–2
 deficiency, 99
 plus progestin, 80
 -dependent neoplasms and COCs, 206
Estrone, 75
Ethinylestradiol, for hirsutism and acne, 47
Ethosuximide, 213–14

European Society for Human Reproduction (ESHRE), 42
Evra, 205–6

F

Fadrozole hydrochloride, for endometriosis, 149
Fallopian tube, 137–8
 surgery to, 139–40
  distal portion occlusion, 140
  intramural/interstitial obstruction, 139
  isthmic/mid-portion occlusion, 139
  results, 140
Falope rings, 271
Familial hirsutism, 56
Female condoms, 188
 advantages, 188
 disadvantages, 189
Female partner
 age, and fertility, 85
 investigation of, 98–9
 ovulatory function, 98–9
Female reproductive system, development of, 5
Ferriman–Gallowey scale, for hirsutism, 54
Fertility, 169
 and age of female partner, 85
 awareness, 176
  background physiology, 176
  lactational amenorrhea method, 177
  methods, advantages of, 177
  ovulation, markers of, 176–7
  postpartum and climacteric period, 177
  problems and disadvantages, 177
 contraceptives
  available methods, effectiveness of, 173, 174
  eligibility criteria for, 175
  ideal contraceptive, features of, 171, 172
 issues, and COCs, 222
 natural regulation of, methods for, 176
 sex and relationships education, 170

 sexually transmitted diseases, 171
Fertility problems
 investigation, 91
 of couple, 92, 93
 of female partner, 98–9
 first -and second-line examinations for, 94
 of male partner, 95–7
 of mechanical factor, possible, 100–11
 management strategies for, 106
 male infertility, 106–7
 mechanical factors in female partner, 108
 ovulatory dysfunction, 107
 unexplained infertility, 108
 management principles for, 104
 prevalence of, 84
Filshie clip, 271
Fimbria, 137
Fimbroplasty, 140
Finasteride
 for acne, 47
 for hirsutism, 47, 59
Fluorescence in situ hybridization (FISH), 165
Flutamide
 for acne, 47
 for hirsutism, 47, 58–9
Folic acid supplementation and conception, relationship between, 86
Follicle-stimulating hormone (FSH), 34
 serum concentration, and PCOS, 46
Follicular development, 37
Follicular phase, 32
Fracture, risk factors of, 79
Frozen embryo transfer replacement cycle (FERC), 161

G

Genes, involved in sex differentiation, 4, 6
Gestational trophoblastic disease, and COCs, 197
Glucocorticoids, 18
Gonadal dysgenesis
 complete, 8
 pure, 8
 mixed, 8
Gonadal failure, and delayed puberty, 29
Gonadal steroid hormones, 21

Gonadorelin, 127
Gonadotropin therapy, for anovulation, 47–8
Gonadotropin deficiency, and delayed puberty, 29
Gonadotropin-releasing hormone (GnRH), 34–5
  agonists, 159–60
    depot vs. daily, 161
    for endometriosis, 149
    for ovulation induction, 71
    protocols, short vs. long, 161
  antagonists, 160–1
Gonadotropins, 128–31
  delivery systems, 128
  FSH-containing preparations, 128
  indications, 128
  monitoring, 130
  multiple pregnancies, prevention of, 131
  ovarian hyperstimulation syndrome, 131
  results, 131, 132
  treatment protocol, 129–30
    conventional, regular protocol, 129
    low-dose step-up protocol, 129–30
    step-down protocol, 130
Gynecology, adolescent, 23

H

Hair growth, distribution of, 99
Hair removal, for hirsutism, 58
Hand–foot–genital (HFG) syndrome, 12
Headaches
  monitoring, and COCs, 221
Health care provider, calculation of pregnancy, 276–7
Hemorrhagic stroke (HS), and COCs, 199
Hermaphroditism, 9
  secondary or pseudohermaphrodites, 9
Hirsutism, 51
  definition of, 52
  differential diagnosis of, 56–7
  etiology of, 55
  history and examination of, 54
  pathophysiology of, 53
  and PCOS, 47
  treatment of, 58
Hormonal analysis
  of hypogonadotropic hypogonadism, 117, 118
  of male, 117, 118
Hormonal examination, 96
Hormone(s), 34–5
  estradiol, 34–5
  follicle-stimulating hormone, 34
  gonadotropin-releasing hormone, 34–5
  levels of ovulatory cycle, 33
  luteinizing hormone, 34
  progesterone, 35
  steroid, 15
Hormone replacement therapy (HRT), 71, 73
  preparations of, 81–2
    oral regimens, 81
    suggested regimens, 81, 82
    transdermal regimens, 81
    vaginal, 81
  risks and benefits of, 80
  side effects and complications of, 81–2
Hot flashes, 76–7
HOX gene, 12
21-hydroxylase deficiency, 9, 57
Hyperandrogenism, 42, 57
Hypergonadotropic hypogonadism, and delayed puberty, 29
Hyperinsulinemia, and PCOS, 44, 46
Hyperprolactinemia, 39, 114
  and amenorrhea, 65
  management of, 71
Hypertension, and COCs, 208
Hypogonadotropic hypogonadism, 63, 114, 128. See also Hypothalamic–pituitary failure
  hormonal analysis of, 117, 118
Hypothalamic–pituitary dysfunction, 38–9
  and amenorrhea, 63–4
  management of, 71–2
  treatment of, 107
Hypothalamic–pituitary failure, 38
  and amenorrhea, 63
  management of, 71
Hypothalamic–pituitary–gonadal axis, 25–6
  in boys, 25–6
  in girls, 25–6
Hypothalamic–pituitary–ovarian axis, 33
Hypothyroidism
  and hyperprolactinemia, 39, 65
Hysterosalpingography (HSG), 105
Hysteroscopy, restoration of endometrial function, 72

I

Idiopathic infertility. See Unexplained infertility
Imaging of testes, 96–7
Imperforate hymen, 72
Implanon, 178
  absolute contraindications for, 244
  bone density concerns in, 237
  contraceptive implant, 240
  timing of insertion, 243
  relative contraindications for, 244
Implantable contraceptives. See Implanon
Infertility, 87. See also Anovulation
  endometriosis-associated, 144
  male, 111
Injectables, 231
  administration, 232
  advantages, 234
  background, 232
  contraindications, 237
  counseling and ongoing supervision, 238
  follow-up, 238
  indications, 234
  mechanism of action and effectiveness, 233–4
  potential drug interactions, 233
  problems and disadvantages, 235–7
  starting routines, 233
In situ conception, and IUDs, 250–1
Insulin
  and PCOS, 44, 46
  resistance, after menopause, 75

Intersex conditions, 7–8
 incidence of, 7
 management of, 8
 presentation and investigation of, 7
Intracytoplasmic sperm injection (ICSI), 106–7, 163, 166
Intrauterine contraception, 247
 copper-bearing devices, 249–54
 levonorgestrel-releasing intrauterine system, 255
 timing of insertions, 259
Intrauterine devices (IUDs), 248
 actinomyces-like organisms, 253
 cancer risk and, 254
 counseling and follow-up, 260
 insertion arrangements, clinical implications for, 252–3
 in emergency contraception cases, 252–3
 with lost threads, 248, 251
 perforation risk of, 251
 PID and, 251–3
Intrauterine insemination (IUI), 106–7, 108, 151
 cost-effectiveness, 154
 indications, 153
 methods, 152
 for mild-factor infertility, 153
 principle, 152
 for unexplained fertility, 153
Investigations, management of, 105
In vitro fertilization (IVF), 108, 108, 155
 for anovulation, 47–8
 assisted reproduction, children born as result of, 166
 complications of, 164
 embryos, number of transferred, 158
 factors affecting outcome of, 157
 intracytoplasmic sperm injection, 163
 metformin in, 127
 oocyte donation, 163
 preimplantationgenetic diagnosis/preimplantationgenetic screening, 165
 procedures during, 159–62
Ischemic stroke (IS), and COCs, 199

L

Lactation, and POP, 224
Lactational amenorrhea method (LAM), 177, 178
 postpartum use, additional methods for, 178
Lamotrigine, 213–14
Lansoprazole, 213–14
Laparoscopic cystectomy, 147
Laparoscopic ovarian drilling (LOD), 133
 for anovulation, 47–8
Laparoscopy, 101, 105, 143, 145–6
Late onset congenital adrenal hyperplasia (LOCAH), 57
Levonorgestrel emergency contraception (LNG-EC), 263
 contraindications, 263
 effectiveness and advantages, 263
 mechanism of action, 263
Levonorgestrel intrauterine system (LNG-IUS), 170, 178, 255, 255
 advantages and indications, 255–6
 contraindications, 257
 established, 258
 relative, 258–9
 counseling, insertion and follow-up, 259, 260
 duration of use in older women, 257
 features of, 256
 infection risk, ectopic pregnancy, future fertility risk, 256
 insertion process, training for, 260
 insertion timing for, 259–60
 method of action and effectiveness, 255
 problems and disadvantages, 256–7
Liver cancer, and COCs, 197, 205–6
Long-acting reversible contraceptives (LARCs), 170, 222, 240
Luteal phase, 32
 support, 162

Luteinizing hormone (LH), 34
 serum concentration, and PCOS, 46
Lybrel, 210–11

M

Male contraception, 181
 coitus interruptus, 182
 condoms, 183
 pill, 184
 vasectomy, 185
Male infertility, 106–7, 111
 etiology of, 113–14
 investigation of, 116
 treatment possibilities for, 106
Male partner, investigation of, 95–7
 examination, 96–7
 history, 96
Mechanical factor infertility, 108
 treatment possibilities for, 108
Medical Eligibility Criteria for Contraceptive Use (WHOMEC), 175
Medications
 and conception, relationship between, 86
 and hyperprolactinemia, 39, 65
Medroxyprogesterone acetate (MPA), 82
 for endometriosis, 148–9
Megestrol, 82
Menarche, 23
Menopause, 73
 alternative treatment, 82
 diagnosing loss of fertility at 278
 hormonal changes, 75
 pathophysiology of, 74
 and POP, 229
 symptoms of, 76–8
 Women's Health Initiative trial, 79
Menorrhagia, and sterilization, 273
Menstrual abnormalities, and injectables, 235
Menstrual bleeding, and POP, 228
Menstrual cycle, 31
Menstrual irregularity, and sterilization, 273
Metformin, 126–7
 for anovulation, 47–8
 dose, 126
 for hirsutism, 47, 58

Metformin (Contd.)
  indications, 126
  in IVF, 127
  mode of action, 126
  for ovulation induction, 71–2
  plus CC, 126–7
  in pregnancy, 127
  side effects, 126
Microsurgical techniques, 139–40, 140
Migraine
  with aura, 208–9
    absolute contraindications, 209
    clinical implications, 209
    features, 209
    relative contraindications, 209–10
  and COCs, 208–10
  differential diagnoses, 210
  and stroke risk, 208
Mineralocorticoids, 18
Mirena. See Levonorgestrel intrauterine system (LNG-IUS)
Mixed antibody reaction (MAR) test, 116
Müllerian anomalies, 10–12
  ASRM classification of, 10–12
Müllerian development, normal, 10
Multifactorial infertility, 106
Multiple pregnancies, 122
  prevention, during ovulation induction, 131

N

National Institute of Child Health and Human Development (NICHD), 42
National Institutes of Health (NIH), 42
Nonoxinol. See Spermicide
Norethindrone, for endometriosis, 148–9
Norethisterone, 82
Normal gonadal–pituitary axis, 117
"No scalpel vasectomy," 274

O

Obesity, 99
  and ovulation induction, 122
  and PCOS, 47

Obstructive male infertility, 113
Occupation and conception, relationship between, 86
Oligomenorrhea, 61
  definition of, 62
  etiology of, 63–6
  investigations of, 67–8, 69
  management of, 70
Oligo-ovulation, 42
  causes of, 38
  treatment possibilities for, 107
Oligospermia, 95–7
Oocyte collection, 162
Oocyte donation, 163
Oral contraceptives (OCs)
  for endometriosis, 148
  for hirsutism and acne, 47
  plus spironolactone, 71–2
Organon, 242
Outflow tract defects
  and amenorrhea, 66
  management of, 71
Ovarian cancer, and sterilization, 273
Ovarian failure, 39, 74
  and amenorrhea, 66
  management of, 71
Ovarian hyperstimulation syndrome (OHSS), 122, 131, 164
  prevention of, 131
Ovarian stimulation, 159–62
  agonists, 159–60
  antagonists, 160–1
  FSH dose selection, 161–2
  LH activity, 161
  monitoring, 162
  protocols, comparison of, 161
  urinary-derived and recombinant gonadotropins, 161–2
Ovary, 36
  carcinomas of, and COCs, 197
  morphology of, 36
  and PCOS, 44
Overweight, 99
Ovulary dysfunction, 107
  treatment possibilities for, 107
Ovulation, 32. See also Anovulation
  induction, 121
    in PCOS women, 49
  markers of, 176–7
Ovulation therapy, 147
Ovum donation, for ovarian failure, 71

P

P450-linked side chain-cleaving enzyme (P450ssc), 18–20
Pain, and IUDs, 254
Pancreatic B-cell function, and PCOS, 44
Pelvic inflammatory disease (PID), 137–8
  and IUDs, 251–3
Peptide hormones, 18
Peritoneum endometriosis, 145
Phasic pills, 210–11
Phytoestrogens, 82
Pill-free intervals, 210–11
Pituitary adenoma
  and hyperprolactinemia, 39, 65
Plasma progesterone concentrations, 98–9
Polycystic ovaries, 42
Polycystic ovary syndrome (PCOS), 41, 56, 63–4, 99
  definition of, 42
  etiology of, 44
  long-term health implications of, 45–6
  management of, 44
  and ovulatory disorders, 38–9
  pathophysiology of, 44
  prevalence of, 43
  women, ovulation induction in, 49
Polymerase chain reaction (PCR), 113
Pomeroy technique, 271
Postcoital contraception, 261
  copper intrauterine devices, 264
  counseling and management, 265–6
  contraception, 265–6
  contraindications, 265
  follow-up, 266
  medical risks, 265
  side effects, 265
  levonorgestrel emergency contraception, 263
Postcoital test (PCT), 96
Postovulatory infertile phase, 176–7
Postpartum period, 177
Precocious onset of puberty, 28
  causes of, 28
Pregnancy. See also Conception

metformin in, 127
status, confirmation of, 276–7
Preimplantation genetic diagnosis (PGD), 165
Preimplantation genetic screening (PGS), 165
Premature menopause, 39, 65
Preovulatory infertile phase, 176–7
Primary amenorrhea, 62, 65
Primary infertility, 88
Primary testicular disease, 113
Progesterone, 16, 35, 2
Progestins, for endometriosis, 148–9
Progestogen-only pill (POP), 178, 223
  absolute contraindications for, 227
  action necessary during full lactation, 224
  advantages and indications, 226
  adverse effects, 225
    nonbleeding, 228
  counselling and ongoing supervision, 228
  and menopause, 229
  monitoring, 229
  return of fertility after, 229
  and drug interactions, 225
  effectiveness, 224
  lactation and, 224
  mechanism of action, 224–5
  missed pills of, 224
  relative contraindications for, 227
  risks and disadvantages, 225
  starting routine for, 228
Progestogens, 81–2
Prolactin-lowering drugs, for hyperprolactinemia, 71
Prolactinoma. See Pituitary adenoma
Propranolol, 82
Proteins, steroid-binding, 22
Proximal tubal disease, 138
Pseudohermaphrodites, 9
Puberty, 24
  delayed onset of, 29
  precocious onset of, 28
  stages of, 27
  Tanner stages of, 27
Pulsatile gonadotropin-releasing hormone therapy, 127

Q
Quick start, 276

R
Rifampicin, 213–14, 225
Rokitansky syndrome, 10–12

S
Saline-infused sonohystogram (SIS), 101
Salpingectomy, 108
Salpingitis isthmica nodosa, 138
Seasonale, 210–1
Secondary amenorrhea, 276–7
  first visit, 276–7
  second visit, 277
Secondary amenorrhea, 62, 65
Secondary infertility, 88
Selected Practice Recommendations for Contraceptive Use (WHOSPR), 175
Selective estrogen receptor modulators (SERMS), 82
Semen analysis, 95–7, 105, 116
  normal and abnormal semen parameters, 116
  WHO reference values for, 95
Serum CA-125 testing, 143
Sex and relationships education (SRE), 170
Sex hormone–binding globulin (SHBG), 75
Sex steroids, conditions affected by and COCs, 206
Sexual differentiation, 3
  genes involved in, 4, 6
  Hand–foot–genital syndrome, 12
  hermaphroditism, 9
  intersex conditions, 7–8
  Müllerian anomalies, 10–12
  SRY gene, 5
  stages of, 4
  Wolffian system, incomplete regression of, 13
Sexually transmitted diseases (STDs), 171
  contract tracing, 171
Skeletal system, and menopause, 77–8
Skin grafting, for transverse vaginal septa, 72
Smoking and conception, relationship between, 86
Society for Assisted Reproductive Technology (SART), 158
Sonohysterography, 101
Sonosalpingography, 101
Spermatogenesis
  causes of failure of, 113
  effect of drugs on, 115
Sperm function tests, 116, 117
Spermicide, 178, 189
  disadvantages, 190
  use for defined populations, 190
Spironolactone
  for acne, 47
  for hirsutism, 47, 58
  plus oral contraceptives, 71–2
SRY (sex-determining region of the Y chromosome) gene, 5
Sterilization, 178, 269, 271
  female, long-term side effects of, 273
    likelihood of regret following, 273
    menstrual irregularity or menorrhagia, 273
    ovarian cancer, 273
    psychological sequelae, 273
  methods, comparison of, 274
  potential reversibility, 272
Steroid hormones, 15, 18
  biosynthesis reactions, 18–20
  gonadal, 21
  steroid-binding proteins, 22
Stress, and hyperprolactinemia, 65
Stroke risk, and migraine, 208
Subarachnoid hemorrhage, and COCs, 199
Surgery
  for endometriosis, 145–6
  to fallopian tube, 139–40
  for hyperprolactinemia, 71

T
Tanner stages of puberty, 27
Teratozoospermia, 95–7
Testosterone, 21, 16, 75
  and hair growth, 53
Thrombophilias, 204

Transient ischemic attacks (TIAs), 210
Transverse vaginal septa, 72
Tubal catheterization, 108
Tubal disorders, 137–8
 anatomy, 137
 pathophysiology, 137–8
 salpingitis isthmica nodosa, 138
Tubal occlusion, 271, 274
Tumor risk, and COCs, 196–8
Turner's syndrome, 39, 99

U

Ultrasound, 101, 143
Unexplained infertility, 108
 treatment possibilities for, 109
Urinary LH kits, 98–9
Urogenital system, and menopause, 77
Uterine disorders, 140
 uterine fibroids, 140

V

Vaginal methods, 187
 caps and diaphragms, 188
 female condoms, 188
 spermicide, 189
Vaginal ring (NuvaRing), 221

Vaginal ultrasound examination, 98–9, 124
Valproate, 213–14
Varicocele, 114
Vasectomy, 185, 271, 274
 failure rates of, 185
Venous thromboembolism (VTE)
 acquired predispositions to, 204
 and COCs, 199, 200–11
 hereditary predispositions to, 204
Venous thrombosis, and HRT, 82
Vigabatrin, 213–14
Virilization, 51

W

Weight loss
 and ovulation, 47–8
 and PCOS, 47, 58, 71–2
Weight-related amenorrhea, 99
Wolffian system, incomplete regression of, 13
Women's Health Initiative (WHI) trial, 79, 80
World Health Organization (WHO)
 classification of amenorrhea and oligomenorrhea, 63–6

classification of anovulation and oligo-ovulation, 38
classification of contraceptives
 contraindications, 175, 172
 eligibility criteria for, 205–11
 absolute contraindications, 205–6
 diabetes mellitus, 207–8
 hypertension, 208
 migraine, 208–10
 pill-free intervals, 210–11
 relative contraindications, 206–7
 reference values for semen analysis, 95

X

X-ray hysterosalpingography (HSG), 100

Y

Yasmin, 219
Y chromosome, 113
YM511
 for endometriosis, 149